Prevention and Control of Infectious Diseases in BRI Countries

Weizhong Yang
Editor

Prevention and Control of Infectious Diseases in BRI Countries

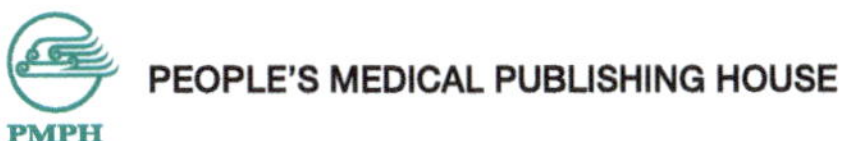

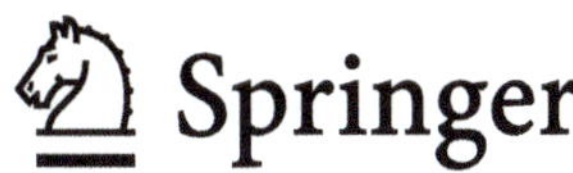

Editor
Weizhong Yang
Chinese Academy of Medical Sciences
& Peking Union Medical College
Chinese Preventive Medicine Association
The UN Consultative Committee on Life
Science and Human Health (CCLH) of
China Association of Science and
Technology (CAST)
Beijing
P.R China

Associate Editors
Xiaofeng Liang
Chinese Preventive Medicine Association
Beijing
P.R China

Huiming Luo
Chinese Center for Disease Control
and Prevention
Beijing
P.R China

Zhongjie Li
Chinese Center for Disease Control
and Prevention
Beijing
P.R China

Luzhao Feng
Chinese Academy of Medical Sciences
& Peking Union Medical College
Beijing
P.R China

Jointly published with People's Medical Publishing House, PR of China

ISBN 978-981-33-6960-3   ISBN 978-981-33-6958-0 (eBook)
https://doi.org/10.1007/978-981-33-6958-0

The print edition is not for sale in China Mainland. Customers from China Mainland please order the print book from: People's Medical Publishing House

This Springer imprint is published by the registered company Springer Nature Singapore Pte Ltd.
The registered company address is: 152 Beach Road, #21-01/04 Gateway East, Singapore 189721, Singapore

Preface

COVID-19 has become the most serious public health emergency since World War II. Virus knows no borders, and epidemic knows no races. Thanks to our painstaking efforts, China has achieved positive results in its fight against the COVID-19 pandemic, effectively safeguarding people's lives and health. At the same time, China is actively engaged in bilateral and multilateral cooperation, unreservedly providing support and assistance to countries in need and sharing experience in prevention, control, and treatment. President Xi Jinping, through summit diplomacy and important events such as the 73rd World Health Assembly and G20 Extraordinary Virtual Leaders' Summit on COVID-19, actively advocates effective international joint prevention and control of COVID-19 and support for international organizations in their efforts. Under the leadership of the National Health Commission, China keeps in touch with countries and health organizations in Africa and Central and Eastern Europe, ASEAN EOC Network, and DG SANTE and frequently exchanges experiences on COVID-19 prevention and control through virtual conferences, which has delivered a positive signal to the world to build a community of common health for mankind, highlighting China's high attention to and support for global health security.

In recent years, outbreaks of avian influenza, Ebola virus disease, Zika virus disease, and cholera have repeatedly alarmed global health security. They not only pose a burden on the economy and society of all countries, but also pose a serious threat to national security, affecting world economic development and social stability. At the 73rd World Health Assembly just held, world leaders called for unity and cooperation in fighting the COVID-19 pandemic, stressing the global sharing of vaccines and medical methods. It is clear that safeguarding global health security has become the most important issue in global governance and an important guarantee for countries to achieve the health-related goals in the 2030 Agenda for Sustainable Development.

Deepening "the Belt and Road" (B&R) health exchanges and cooperation and building the Silk Road of Health Cooperation will not only help implement the Healthy China initiative, but also contribute to the public health security of B&R countries. In November 2018, the National Health Commission stated in the *Circular on the Issuance of Guidelines on Advancing "the Belt and Road" Health Exchanges and Cooperation (2018–2022)* that it is necessary to deepen exchanges and cooperation with B&R countries in the field of epidemic prevention and control, effectively guard against the threat of infectious diseases, and provide a solid health security guarantee for facilities connectivity, unimpeded trade, and population movements.

In view of the significance of strengthening international cooperation in the prevention and treatment of infectious diseases to "the Belt and Road" initiative, the Chinese Preventive Medicine Association (CPMA), with the support of the China Association for Science and Technology, organized experts to consult the websites of international organizations such as the WHO, UNICEF, GOARN, ProMED USAID, and Greater Mekong Subregion (GMS), websites of national health administration departments, CDCs and relevant technical support departments, and databases of scientific papers, such as Wanfang, CNKI, PubMed, and Medline to widely collect scientific and technological literature and academic works and systematically assess the risk of 21 major infectious diseases threatening B&R countries (cholera, polio, measles, meningitis, Japanese encephalitis, diphtheria, hepatitis A, tuberculosis, influenza, dengue fever, Zika virus disease, yellow fever, chikungunya, Rift Valley fever, plague, malaria, Ebola virus disease, MERS, schistoso-miasis, COVID-19 and AIDS), so as to provide decision support for international cooperation among B&R countries in the field of epidemic prevention and control in the future. This book consists of 14 chapters. Chapter 1 is an overview. Chapter 2 introduces the history of health cooperation between China and other B&R countries. Chapters 3–14 introduce the prevalence of major infectious diseases threatening B&R countries such as cholera, vaccine preventable diseases (polio, measles, meningitis, Japanese encephalitis, diphtheria, and hepatitis A), tuberculosis, influenza, and insect-borne diseases (dengue fever, Zika virus disease, yellow fever, chikungunya, and Rift Valley fever), plague, malaria, Ebola virus disease, MERS, schistosomiasis, COVID-19 and AIDS, risk factors, and principles and cases of their prevention and control.

Because of the tight schedule for soliciting and compiling contributions, and most data relying on secondary source materials, there are inevitably omissions and even errors in this book. We sincerely hope that you will point out them.

Beijing, People's Republic of China Weizhong Yang

Acknowledgments

Sincere thanks should be extended to the National Health Commission, China Association for Science and Technology, and the Chinese Center for Disease Control and Prevention that has supported the preparation of this book. All the authors of this book and Dr. Chin-Kei Lee who checked and polished the text of this book, in particular, are appreciated for their hard work. Thanks to People's Medical Publishing House (WHO Health Information and Publishing Cooperation Center) for coordinating the publication work. It is all of your selfless dedication that has guaranteed the scheduled publication of the book.

Contents

Contributors

Xuhong Ding Chinese Center for Disease Control and Prevention, Beijing, People's Republic of China

Luzhao Feng Chinese Academy of Medical Sciences & Peking Union Medical College, Beijing, People's Republic of China

Xiaoxia Huang National Institute for Viral Disease Control and Prevention, China CDC, Beijing, People's Republic of China

Biao Kan National Institute for Communicable Diseases Control and Prevention, China CDC, Beijing, People's Republic of China

Chao Li Chinese Center for Disease Control and Prevention, Beijing, People's Republic of China

Jiandong Li National Institute for Viral Disease Control and Prevention, China CDC, Beijing, People's Republic of China

Qun Li Chinese Center for Disease Control and Prevention, Beijing, People's Republic of China

Wei Li National Institute for Communicable Diseases Control and Prevention, China CDC, Beijing, People's Republic of China

Zhongjie Li Chinese Center for Disease Control and Prevention, Beijing, People's Republic of China

Xiaofeng Liang Chinese Preventive Medicine Association, Beijing, People's Republic of China

Fengfeng Liu Chinese Center for Disease Control and Prevention, Beijing, People's Republic of China

Huiming Luo Chinese Center for Disease Control and Prevention, Beijing, People's Republic of China

Guijun Ning Chinese Center for Disease Control and Prevention, Beijing, People's Republic of China

Yingjun Qian National Institute of Parasitic Diseases, China CDC, Shanghai, People's Republic of China

Xiaona Shen National Institute for Communicable Diseases Control and Prevention, China CDC, Beijing, People's Republic of China

Qiru Su Chinese Center for Disease Control and Prevention, Beijing, People's Republic of China

Xiaoqi Wang Chinese Center for Disease Control and Prevention, Beijing, People's Republic of China

Yali Wang Chinese Center for Disease Control and Prevention, Beijing, People's Republic of China

Wei Wu National Institute for Viral Disease Control and Prevention, China CDC, Beijing, People's Republic of China

Caihong Xu Chinese Center for Disease Control and Prevention, Beijing, People's Republic of China

Weizhong Yang Chinese Academy of Medical Sciences & Peking Union Medical College, Chinese Preventive Medicine Association, The UN Consultative Committee on Life Science and Human Health (CCLH) of China Association of Science and Technology (CAST), Beijing, P.R China

Chuchu Ye Shanghai Pudong New Area Center for Disease Control and Prevention, Shanghai, People's Republic of China

Heya Yi Chinese Preventive Medicine Association, Beijing, People's Republic of China

Guang Zhang National Center for AIDS/STD Control and Prevention, China CDC, Beijing, People's Republic of China

Hui Zhang Chinese Center for Disease Control and Prevention, Beijing, People's Republic of China

Jiandong Zheng Chinese Center for Disease Control and Prevention, Beijing, People's Republic of China

Sheng Zhou Chinese Center for Disease Control and Prevention, Beijing, People's Republic of China

Xiaonong Zhou National Institute of Parasitic Diseases, China CDC, Shanghai, People's Republic of China

Abbreviations

AFP	acute flaccid paralysis
AIDS	acquired immunodeficiency syndrome
APEC	Asia-Pacific Economic Cooperation
ARDS	acute respiratory distress syndrome
ASEAN EOC Network	Association of Southeast Asian Nations Emergency Operations Centre Network for Public Health Emergencies
B&R	the Belt and Road
bOPV	bivalent oral polio vaccine
BRI	Belt and Road Initiative
BRICS	Brazil, Russia, India, China and South Africa
CCA	circulating cathodic antigen
CD4 cells	CD4+T lymphocytes
CDC	Centers for Disease Control and Prevention
CFR	case fatality rate
China CDC	Chinese Center for Disease Control and Prevention
CHIKV	chikungunya virus
CNIC	Chinese National Influenza Center
CNKI	China National Knowledge Infrastructure
COVID-19	coronavirus disease 2019
CoVs	coronaviruses
CRE	carbapenem-resistant Enterobacteriaceae
CRFs	recombinant forms
cVDPV	circulating vaccine-derived polioviruses
DENV	dengue virus
DEWS	Disease Early Warning System
DG SANTE	Directorate General for Health and Food Safety
DOTS	directly observed therapy
DRC	Democratic Republic of Congo
EBOV-B	Bundibugyo Ebola virus
EBOV-R	Reston Ebola virus
EBOV-S	Sudan Ebola virus
EBOV-TF	Tai Forest Ebola virus

EBOV-Z	Zaire Ebola virus
ECSA	East Central South Africa
EMA	European Medicines Agency
EOC	Emergency Operations Centre
EPI	Expanded Programme on Immunization
EVD	Ebola virus disease
EYE	Eliminate Yellow Fever Epidemics
FDA	Food and Drug Administration
GAVI	The Global Alliance for Vaccines and Immunisation
GBS	Guillain-Barré syndrome
GISRS	Global Influenza Surveillance and Response System
GOARN	Global Outbreak Alert and Response Network
GTFCC	Global Task Force on Cholera Control
HAART	highly active antiretroviral therapy
HIV	human immunodeficiency virus
ICG	International Coordinating Group
ICU	intensive care unit
IDSRS	Integrated Disease Surveillance and Response System
IFRC	International Federation of Red Cross and Red Crescent Societies
IHR	International Health Regulation
IMS	incident management system
IPV	inactivated polio vaccine
IRAT	Influenza Risk Assessment Tool
JE	Japanese encephalitis
LGAs	Local government areas
MCH	maternal and child health
MDA	mass drug administration
MDR/RR-TB	multiple drugs resistant tuberculosis
MDR-TB	multidrug-resistant TB
MERS	Middle East respiratory syndrome
MERS-CoV	Middle East respiratory syndrome coronavirus
MMT	methadone maintenance treatment
MMWR	Morbidity and Mortality Weekly Report
MOU	memorandum of understanding
MSF	Médecins Sans Frontières
MSM	men who have sex with men
nPEP	nonoccupational post-exposure prophylaxis
NPIs	non-pharmaceutic interventions
NTDs	neglected tropical diseases
OPV	oral polio vaccine
PBM	pediatric bacterial meningitis
PC	preventive chemotherapy
PCR	polymerase chain reaction
PFGE	pulsed field gel electrophoresis

PITC	provider-initiated HIV testing and counseling
PLWH	people living with HIV
PMVCs	Yellow Fever Preventive Mass Vaccination Campaigns
Polio	Poliomyelitis
PrEP	pre-exposure prophylaxis
PROMED	Program for Monitoring Emerging Diseases
R_0	basic regeneration index
RR-TB	rifampicin resistant tuberculosis
RVFV	Rift Valley fever virus
SAC	school-age children
SARS	severe acute respiratory syndrome
SARS-Cov	SARS coronavirus
SBM	Swachh Bharat Mission
SCH	schistosomiasis
SDB	safc and dignified burial
SIA	supplementary immunization activity
SMS	short message service
SNPs	single-nucleotide polymorphisms
SOPs	standard operating procedures
STD	sexually transmitted disease
STH	soil-transmitted helminthiasis
TB	tuberculosis
tOPV	trivalent oral polio vaccine
TST	tuberculin susceptibility test
UK	United Kingdom
UNAIDS	Joint United Nations Programme on HIV/AIDS
UNICEF	United Nations International Children's Emergency Fund
UNMEER	United Nations Mission for Ebola Emergency Response
US	United States
USAID	United States Agency for International Development
V. cholerae	*Vibrio cholerae*
VCT	voluntary counseling and testing
WA	West Africa
WBC	white blood cell
WER	Weekly Epidemiological Record
WHA	World Health Assembly
WHO	World Health Organization
WPV1	wild poliovirus type 1
WPV2	wild poliovirus type 2
WPV3	wild poliovirus type 3
Y. pestis	*Yersinia pestis*
YFV	yellow fever virus
ZIKV	Zika virus
2019-nCoV	2019 novel coronavirus

Introduction

1

Heya Yi, Chuchu Ye, and Weizhong Yang

1.1 Significance of the "Belt and Road Initiative"

1.1.1 Proposal and Development of the "Belt and Road Initiative"

In September and October 2013, during a visit to Central and Southeast Asia, President Xi Jinping proposed an important initiative to jointly construct the "Silk Road Economic Belt" and the "Twenty-First Century Maritime Silk Road" (hereinafter referred to as the "Belt and Road Initiative") [1]. His proposal aroused the immediate attention of the international community. Availing itself of the historic symbolism of the ancient "Silk Road" and under the banner of peaceful development, the "Belt and Road Initiative" aims to actively develop economic cooperation partnerships with countries neighboring the project's routes while building a community of shared interests, futures, and responsibilities based on mutual political trust, economic integration, and cultural inclusiveness [2]. On March 28, 2015, the

The original version of this chapter was revised. A correction to this chapter is available at https://doi.org/10.1007/978-981-33-6958-0_15

H. Yi
Chinese Preventive Medicine Association, Beijing, People's Republic of China

C. Ye
Shanghai Pudong New Area Center for Disease Control and Prevention, Shanghai, People's Republic of China

W. Yang (✉)
Chinese Academy of Medical Sciences & Peking Union Medical College, Chinese Preventive Medicine Association, The UN Consultative Committee on Life Science and Human Health (CCLH) of China Association of Science and Technology (CAST), Beijing, P.R China
e-mail: yangwz@chinacdc.cn

W. Yang (ed.), *Prevention and Control of Infectious Diseases in BRI Countries*, https://doi.org/10.1007/978-981-33-6958-0_1

National Development and Reform Commission, the Ministry of Foreign Affairs and the Ministry of Commerce of the People's Republic of China issued "Vision and Actions of Jointly Building the Silk Road Economic Belt and the Twenty-First Century Maritime Silk Road." In an effort to clarify the "Belt and Road Initiative," this document elaborates on the project's historical context, principle of joint construction, logical framework, cooperative focus and cooperation mechanism, among other aspects. Based on a fundamental position of "policy coordination, connectivity of infrastructure and facilities, unimpeded trade, financial integration and people-to-people bonds," the document highlights the goals of promoting economic prosperity and regional economic cooperation among countries along the "Belt and Road," strengthening exchange and mutual learning among different civilizations, promoting world peace and development, and benefiting the people of all countries [2].

1.1.2 Significance of the "Belt and Road Initiative"

The "Belt and Road Initiative" is China's most important initiative for regional cooperation and a form of economic diplomacy involving the investment of a wide variety of resources. The project reflects China's needs for comprehensively deepening reform and opening up to the outside world and will serve the fundamental interests of all participating parties. It adheres to the concepts of joint discussion, joint construction, and mutual benefit and aims to achieve win–win cooperation in terms of communal development and common prosperity [3, 4].

1.1.3 China and Countries Along the Belt and Road

The "Belt and Road" will extend across Asia, Europe, and Africa. On one end is the energetic East Asia economic circle, while on the other lies the developed European economic circle. In between are the vast hinterland countries that hold great potential for economic development. The "Silk Road Economic Belt" seeks to create uninterrupted transport links between China and Europe (the Baltic Sea) via Central Asia and Russia, between China and the Persian Gulf and the Mediterranean through Central and West Asia, and between China and Southeast Asia, South Asia, and the Indian Ocean. The "Twenty-First Century Maritime Silk Road" is proposed to extend from China's coastal ports across the South China Sea to the Indian Ocean, Europe, and the South Pacific [5].

This book uses the following criteria in selecting 34 "Belt and Road" countries as key research objects: the existence of an intergovernmental framework of cooperation with China, close economic ties and frequent exchanges of governmental personnel with China, broad space for development, as well as medical and health cooperation needs and prospects, in particular, in terms of weakness in preventing and treating certain infectious diseases because of the influence of traditional religious, cultural, and social customs. In the Asia Pacific region, countries selected are Mongolia, Singapore, Malaysia, Thailand, Indonesia, the Philippines, Brunei,

Cambodia, Myanmar, Laos and Vietnam. In Central Asia, they are Kazakhstan, Uzbekistan, Turkmenistan, Tajikistan, and Kyrgyzstan. In West Asia, they are Iran, Iraq, Turkey, Israel, Saudi Arabia, and the United Arab Emirates. In South Asia, they are Afghanistan, Pakistan, India, Bangladesh, Sri Lanka, the Maldives, and Nepal. In Eastern Europe, they are Russia and Ukraine. Finally, in Africa, they are Kenya, Ethiopia, and Egypt.

1.2 Significance of Health Cooperation in the "Belt and Road Initiative"

1.2.1 Overview of Health Cooperation Between Countries Along the "Belt and Road" and China

Partial statistics in recent years have shown that China has worked closely in the health field with countries along the "Belt and Road" [6]. China has signed bilateral intergovernmental health cooperation agreements or memoranda of understanding with Mongolia, the Philippines, Laos, Cambodia, Malaysia, Myanmar, Singapore, Thailand, Brunei, Vietnam, Indonesia, Pakistan, Nepal, Maldives, Bangladesh, Sri Lanka, India, Afghanistan, Saudi Arabia, Turkey, Iran, Israel, Kazakhstan, Kyrgyzstan, Tajikistan, Turkmenistan, Uzbekistan, Russia, Ukraine, Egypt, and other countries. The cooperation covers human resources development in the health field, including health management, the health of women and children, the prevention and control of infectious and chronic diseases, health education, clinical diagnosis, and treatment technology, as well as medical and health services. In addition to bilateral cooperation through exchanges and cooperation platforms (including World Health Organization (WHO) multilateral mechanisms, the Forum on China-Africa Health Cooperation, the China-ASEAN Health Cooperation Forum, the China-CEEC Health Ministers' Forum, the China-Arab States Health Cooperation Forum, the BRICS Health Ministers Meeting, the Meeting of Health Ministers of the Shanghai Cooperation Organization, the G20 Health Ministers' Meeting, the Lancang-Mekong Cooperation program, the Greater Mekong Subregion program and the APEC Health Working Group), China and the "Belt and Road" countries are comprehensively increasing health cooperation and jointly seeking to safeguard regional health and security through various formats, such as high-level mutual visits, institutional exchange and dialogue, cooperative projects, and cooperation agreements.

1.2.2 Health Cooperation in the "Belt and Road Initiative"

Health cooperation, with the aim of improving people's health and well-being, is an area of cooperation with low political sensitivity and high social recognition [7]. It is not only an important aspect of international policy coordination but also a significant link to connect people. Deepening "Belt and Road" health exchanges and cooperation and constructing a "Silk Road" for health are important to a healthy

China and represent a popular foundation and strong argument for the "Belt and Road Initiative," as well as a requirement in building a community with a shared human future. In October 2015, the "Three-year Plan for the Implementation of the 'Belt and Road Initiative' Health Exchange and Cooperation (2015–2017)" was published by the former National Health and Family Planning Commission, and the efforts to realize a healthy "Silk Road" have yielded preliminary results. In January 2017, President Xi Jinping visited WHO headquarters. The Government of the People's Republic of China and the World Health Organization signed the "Memorandum of Understanding" on Cooperation in the Health Field of the "Belt and Road" a milestone in the cooperation between the two sides to improve the health of countries along the "Belt and Road." In November 2018, the National Health Commission published "Guidelines for Further Promoting the 'Belt and Road Initiative' for Health Cooperation and Exchange," which clarified cooperation in key areas of strengthening health safety and promoting health development and innovation.

1.2.3 Main Components of Health Cooperation in the "Belt and Road Initiative"

The primary components of health cooperation and exchange are as follows: strengthening the prevention and control of infectious diseases and the construction of a health emergency response capacity, enhancing the health system, promoting women and children's health, improving healthcare services and management, boosting the development of traditional medicine, promoting healthy aging, furthering the prevention and control of chronic diseases, advancing medical technology, research, development, and developing the health industry [7]. Health cooperation and exchanges have strengthened health security and public support for the "Belt and Road Initiative."

1.3 Infectious Diseases Remaining an Important Public Health Security Problem

1.3.1 Dual Threats of New and Old Infectious Diseases and the Transnational and Transcontinental Transmission of These Diseases [8–10]

In the last 40 years, the world has been faced with the dual threats of new and old infectious diseases, seeing a resurgence, due to natural disasters, ecological changes, wars, weakened public health systems, etc., of many ancient infectious diseases brought under control in the past.

A few months after the 2010 earthquake in Haiti, the largest cholera outbreak ever occurred in a single country after the twentieth century sickened more than 680,000 Haitians, killing more than 8000.

In 2002, Tajikistan announced the eradication of polio. However, from February to July 2010, Tajikistan saw an outbreak of wild poliovirus type 1 (originated in India). A total of 458 cases of wild poliovirus were reported across 35 administrative regions, causing the death of 26 people. Subsequently, the epidemic spread to three other polio-free countries: Russia (14 cases), Turkmenistan (3 cases), and Kazakhstan (1 case). The WHO Western Pacific Region, which includes China, was declared polio-free in 2000. However, an outbreak caused by an imported poliovirus occurred in 2011 in Xinjiang. WHO confirmed that it had been caused by a wild-type poliovirus imported from Pakistan, as evidence showed a high degree of homologous nucleotide sequencing in the viruses isolated in Hotan and in Pakistan. In recent years, Pakistan and Afghanistan faced domestic sustained circulation of WPV1 and VDPV outbreak, especially in the first half of the year 2020, both WPV1 cases and type 2 VDPV cases number reached the highest level compared with the same period during 2016–2019, as 55 WPV1 and 52 VDPV2 in Pakistan, 26 WPV1 and 29 VDPV2 cases in Afghanistan, which are signals of importation and wide-spread of polio-virus to other countries. Type 2 VDPV is becoming as risk as wild polio-virus after the SWITCH of polio vaccine from trivalent OPV to bivalent OPV, disposing of type 2 component in OPV vaccine, population's susceptibility to type 2 polio is increasing.

In October 2017, the largest outbreak of hepatitis A in the United States in the last 20 years sickened more than 600 individuals and resulted in more than 20 deaths.

Since the beginning of the twentieth century, tuberculosis (TB) has been brought under control in many countries. However, since the late 1980s, many developed and developing countries have experienced a sharp rise in TB to the extent that the WHO declared a global TB emergency in 1993. Today, the incidence of TB in many parts of the world remains high, and outbreaks continue to occur in certain areas. The medication resistance and ongoing transmission of *Mycobacterium tuberculosis* remain a serious challenge worldwide.

In 1997, the world's first human case of the highly pathogenic avian influenza virus H5N1 was observed in China's Hong Kong Special Administrative Region. Subsequent human avian influenza H5N1 outbreaks occurred in many countries in East Asia, Southeast Asia, and North Africa, all with high mortality. In March 2013, acute respiratory infections caused by the new H7N9 avian influenza virus were first detected in Shanghai, China. From 2013 to 2017, the H7N9 avian influenza cases reached more than 1000, and the mortality was also high. In the spring of 2009, an H1N1 influenza pandemic that began in Mexico and the United States spread to 214 countries, territories, and regions in less than a year, causing tens of millions of cases and 18,449 deaths. Another more than 200,000 died from associated respiratory diseases.

Zika virus disease was listed by WHO as "a public health emergency of international concern" from February to November 2016 and received much attention. Before 2007, the distribution of Zika virus disease was mainly limited to tropical Africa and Southeast Asia. However, outbreaks were reported in Pacific countries from 2013 to 2014. After Zika virus disease was reported in Brazil in 2015, the disease spread rapidly. As of 2017, vector transmission of Zika virus disease had been found in 84 countries. Over the past 50 years, the reported incidence of dengue fever has increased 30-fold and is endemic or highly endemic in 128 tropical and subtropical countries in Asia, the Americas, Africa, and Europe. According to estimates, 390 million individuals worldwide are infected with dengue fever annually, among whom 96 million are severe incidences. Yellow fever was formerly endemic in tropical regions of Central and South America and Africa, with no cases reported in Asia. Angola has been overwhelmed with a widespread yellow fever epidemic since December 2015. As of the end of 2016, yellow fever had killed at least 376 individuals and spread to surrounding countries, causing at least 16 deaths in the Democratic Republic of the Congo. Since 2016, China has reported more than ten imported yellow fever cases from abroad. Rift Valley fever has been detected in more than 30 countries. The disease is mainly distributed in Eastern and Southern Africa, including Kenya, Zimbabwe, Zambia, Namibia, and Somalia. Outbreaks have also occurred in Saudi Arabia and Yemen in Asia. In 2016, the first case of imported Rift Valley fever was detected in China.

In August 2017, the plague outbreak in Madagascar, with more than 2000 cases and over 200 deaths, was the strongest in 50 years and arose widespread global concern.

In addition, over the last 40 years, new infectious disease pathogens or their corresponding diseases have appeared nearly every year worldwide, some of which have developed into widespread epidemics. Since the 1970s, repeated outbreaks of Ebola have occurred in Africa. In December 2013, an outbreak of Ebola began in Guinea in West Africa and later spread to other West African countries, such as Liberia, Sierra Leone, and Nigeria. This West African Ebola outbreak resulted in the highest recorded number of incidences and deaths and was the most widespread. WHO attached substantial importance to the outbreak, announcing on August 8, 2014, that the epidemic was "unusual" and constituted an "international public health emergency." In February 2003, severe acute respiratory syndrome (SARS) caused by SARS coronavirus (SARS-Cov) was first detected in China. It spread rapidly around the world and caused more than 8000 infections in 29 countries (mainly adults aged 25–70 years) and more than 700 deaths. No case has been reported since 2005.

In September 2012, cases of Middle East Respiratory Syndrome (MERS) were first detected in Saudi Arabia, and subsequent cases of MERS were reported in several countries in Asia, Africa, Europe, and the Americas. In May 2015, after several imported cases found in South Korea, there was a clustered MERS outbreak. A total of 186 confirmed cases were reported, of which 36 were fatal. Two of these confirmed cases might be infections within a family, and the remaining ones were infections occurred in medical- and healthcare-related locations. There was one case of initial incidence, 29 second-generation cases, 125 third-generation cases, 25 fourth-generation cases, and six cases of unknown generation. With the exception of the initial incidence, secondary cases occurred in 12 cases, of which one case resulted in 84 subsequent infections. In late May 2015, a case of MERS imported from South Korea was found in Guangdong Province, China. Thanks to its effective public health measures, there were no second-generation cases.

In December 2019, pneumonia of unknown cases occurred in Wuhan City, Hubei Province, China. Laboratory tests revealed that it was caused by a novel coronavirus, which was later named 2019 Novel coronavirus (2019-nCoV) by the WHO. It caused a pandemic in 2020, and the pandemic continued to spread. According to the latest WHO epidemic report, as of CET, 1 November 2020, a total of 45,942,902 confirmed cases have been reported in 217 countries and regions on six continents, with a total of 1,192,644 deaths, and a death/case ratio of 2.6%.

In the 1980s, acquired immunodeficiency syndrome (AIDS) was first discovered in the United States. Then it spread worldwide and became a serious public health problem.

1.3.2 Risk Factors for Infectious Disease Transmission

Modern transportation has facilitated the movement of people and things around the world. There are approximately 5000 airports worldwide, with one million flights per week and approximately four billion trips per year. Pathogens do not require visas to travel freely, and thus, the transport system poses risks with respect to disease transmission. Both SARS and MERS were spread rapidly across borders and continents in a short period of time by travelers. Deforestation, large-scale dam construction, mining, oil and natural gas projects, global warming caused by CO_2 emissions, and changes in the ecological environment have all affected the distribution of pathogens and vector organisms, giving rise to the increased incidence or distribution changes in mosquito-borne dengue fever and Zika virus disease and increased risk with respect to water-borne diseases, like cholera. Natural disasters and accidents undermine the effect of safeguard measures for public health, like the water supply system, hence the outbreaks of infectious diseases. As war, natural disasters, and other factors weaken or even destroy the healthcare system, diseases once brought under control may regain virulence, and as a result, measures taken to eradicate the disease have to be adopted once again, like in the polio outbreak.

Unsafe blood, biological products, and medical practices due to regulatory failure or accidents can facilitate the transmission and even outbreak of iatrogenic disease. The outbreak of SARS in 2003 in China and MERS in 2015 in South Korea both involved high rates of hospital transmission, which caused substantial socioeconomic losses and social panic.

The misuse of antibiotics in humans, poultry, and livestock leads to antibiotic resistance and the spread of pathogens, which can increase the risk of infectious diseases. In the past 10 years, many countries have reported cases of carbapenem-resistant Enterobacteriaceae (CRE) infection, and this infection has exhibited a trend of rapid increase. Pressure from the environment and the host causes the pathogenic microorganisms to mutate such that nonpathogenic strains become pathogenic, and weakly virulent strains become strongly virulent, or new pathogenic strains.

In 2001, an incident involving white anthrax powder occurred in the United States. Biological terrorism represents another potential source of outbreaks of infectious diseases.

Before the total elimination of original risk factors for infectious diseases, new ones have emerged. Risk factors for infectious diseases are widespread. As a result, new infectious diseases have emerged continuously before the eradication of ancient ones. Coupled with people's limited understanding of infectious disease pathogens and their epidemic patterns, the occurrence and development of infectious diseases remain highly uncertain. The prevention and control of infectious diseases remains a very challenging task and must not be neglected. In implementing the "Belt and Road Initiative," it is necessary and important to thoroughly assess the risk of infectious diseases and adopt corresponding countermeasures.

1.4 Data Sources

This book uses data from the World Health Organization (WHO), United Nations International Children's Emergency Fund (UNICEF), Global Outbreak Alert and Response Network (GOARN), websites of international organizations such as ProMED, USAID, Greater Mekong communique, websites of national health administration departments and CDCs from several counties, domestic and international databases of scientific and technological papers, such as Wanfang, CNKI, PubMed, MEDLINE, etc. Relevant websites are as follows:

- http://www.fmprc.gov.cn/web/
- http://www.who.int/countries/en/
- http://www.who.int/topics/zh/
- http://www.who.int/gho/countries/en/
- http://www.who.int/immunization/monitoring_surveillance/data/en/
- http://www.who.int/ith/en/
- http://219.238.166.215/mcp/index.asp
- http://www.healthdata.org/gbd
- http://www.healthmap.org/zh/
- http://www.oecd.org/health/
- http://wwwnc.cdc.gov/travel

References

1. People's Daily Online. Carry forward the friendship among peoples and create a better future together. http://www.people.com.cn/24hour/n/2013/0908/c25408-22842973.html. Accessed 8 Sep 2013.
2. People's Daily Online. Xi Jinping addressed the Indonesian Parliament: Work together to build a China-ASEAN community of shared future. http://politics.people.com.cn/n/2013/1003/c1024-23101573.html. Accessed 3 Oct 2013.
3. Ge S. Global vision—"the Belt and Road". Int Stud. 2016;2:1–13.
4. Guoyou S. The strategic vision of "the Belt and Road" and new development of China's economic diplomacy. Collected papers of Division of International Studies. Chin Acad Soc Sci. 2017;10:255–67.

5. The vision and actions of jointly building the Silk Road Economic Belt and the 21st Century Maritime Silk Road. [N/OL]. Xinhuanet. Accessed 6 Apr 2015.
6. Siling Y. Governance and challenges of China's relations with countries along the Belt and Road. South Asian Studies. 2015;2:15–34.
7. Hongwei Y. Build a silk road of health in the context of the Belt and Road Initiative. China Health. 2016;7:40–1.
8. China Preventive Medicine Association. Report on disciplinary development in Public Health and Preventive Medicine 2016–2017. Beijing: China Science and Technology Press, 2018.
9. Weizhong Y. China's Health Emergency Response 2003–2013. Beijing: People's Medical Publishing House; 2014.
10. China Preventive Medicine Association. Report on disciplinary development in Public Health and Preventive Medicine 2014–2015. Beijing: China Science and Technology Press; 2016.

2 Health Cooperation Between China and Other "Belt and Road" Countries

Xuhong Ding and Xiaoqi Wang

2.1 East Asia

China and Mongolia have close cooperation partnership in the area of health. The governments of the two countries signed an agreement on health cooperation in the 1990s and have signed a series of 5-year health cooperation work plans since 2004. In August 2017, the two countries renewed another 5-year health cooperation workplan (2017–2021). There were frequent bilateral ministerial visits in the health sector. Health cooperation between China and Mongolia mainly focuses on traditional medicine, infectious disease control and prevention, and healthcare services. The achievements made included the training of human resources in clinical medicine and public health, medical technology communication and exchange, the establishment of medical facilities and channels for Mongolian patients to obtain medical treatment in China. The two countries also cooperate under multilateral mechanisms, such as the Central Asian Regional Economic Cooperation (CAREC) mechanism, WHO multilateral mechanism, etc.

2.2 Southeast Asia

The ten member states of the Association of Southeast Asian Nations (ASEAN), including Philippines, Cambodia, Laos, Malaysia, Myanmar, Singapore, Thailand, Brunei, Vietnam and Indonesia, have cooperated well with China in the health sector. All ten ASEAN member states have signed bilateral intergovernmental health cooperation agreements or Memorandums of Understanding (MOU) with China.

X. Ding · X. Wang (✉)
Chinese Center for Disease Control and Prevention, Beijing, People's Republic of China
e-mail: wangxq@chinacdc.cn

W. Yang (ed.), *Prevention and Control of Infectious Diseases in BRI Countries*,
https://doi.org/10.1007/978-981-33-6958-0_2

China and six ASEAN member states, that is, Cambodia, Laos, Malaysia, Singapore, Thailand and Brunei, have frequent ministerial-level visits and exchanges in health. Infectious disease control and prevention is a common concern all ASEAN countries share with China. Except for Vietnam, the other nine countries also focus on traditional medicine in their work with China. The priorities differ with conditions of each country and mainly include human resources development in health, health management, maternal and child health (MCH), noncommunicable disease (NCD) control and prevention, food and drug safety, health education, the technology of clinical diagnosis and treatment, medical service provision, etc.

Most of the health cooperation between China and ASEAN countries are undertaken with the support of bilateral or regional funds mainly invested by the Chinese government, as well as under the traditional or new multilateral cooperation mechanisms, such as the ASEAN plus China, Japan, South Korea (10+3) Cooperation Mechanism, "China-ASEAN Health Cooperation Forum" and its Joint Declaration, Greater Mekong Subregional (GMS) Cooperation Mechanism, Lancang-Mekong Cooperation Mechanism, Asia-Pacific Economic Cooperation (APEC) Mechanism, and WHO multilateral mechanism. The cooperation is committed to promoting in-depth communication and exchanges among health professionals, enhancing the capacity building of institutes responsible for infectious disease control and prevention in ASEAN countries, establishing regional infectious disease surveillance and emergency response mechanisms, and jointly maintaining regional health security.

2.3 South Asia

China has signed bilateral intergovernmental MOU on health cooperation with three of the six South Asian countries (Bangladesh, India, Maldives, Nepal, Pakistan and Sri Lanka), that is, Pakistan, Maldives and India. The governments of Nepal and China have signed the "Protocol on the Dispatch of A Medical Team from China to Serve in Nepal." Bangladesh and Sri Lanka have not signed any intergovernmental health cooperation agreements or MOU with China.

Pakistan and India have built up relatively good partnership with China in the health sector. Pakistan and China have frequent exchanges of high-level visits of health officials. In the past, Pakistan assisted China in fighting against SARS and supported China during Sichuan earthquake in 2008. China also sent public health experts to Pakistan for polio elimination. The high-level health officials of India and China have exchanged visits many times, and the governments of the two countries have actively worked together in promoting the institutionalization of the ministerial conference and population development within the framework of BRICS, and advocating the realization of the Sustainable Development Goals (SDG), as well as the Millennium Development Goals (MDG) under South-South cooperation. As Nepal and China share borders, the two countries have cooperated relatively more closely in health. The Chinese government has provided steady health assistance to Nepal, including dispatching a medical team to serve in Nepal, providing healthcare services to Nepal national leaders and sending medical teams to conduct emergency rescue and disposal after earthquakes in Nepal.

Since the "Belt and Road" initiative was launched in 2013, China has strengthened its health cooperation and partnership with South Asian countries and meanwhile, new cooperation models have been explored and developed. The needs and willingness of health cooperation between the six South Asian countries and China are strengthened. China has progressively advanced its collaboration with Pakistan on traditional medicine, and gradually furthered its health cooperation with India in the framework of BRICS. In 2016, the ministers of Health of Nepal, Maldives, and Bangladesh visited China, and Vice Minister of the National Health and Family Planning Commission of China visited Sri Lanka. In September 2014, China and Maldives signed intergovernmental MOU on health cooperation. In 2016, China sent ophthalmologists to Maldives and Sri Lanka on the "Bright Journey—Eye Care Mission." In 2015 and 2016, China hosted Bangladesh-China-India-Myanmar Cooperation Forum on Health and Disease Control under the framework of Bangladesh-China-India-Myanmar regional cooperation and Bangladesh representatives joined the meetings.

2.4 West Asia

Of the seven West Asian countries, including Afghanistan, the UAE, Saudi Arabia, Turkey, Iran, Iraq and Israel, except for the UAE and Iraq, all other countries have signed bilateral intergovernmental health agreements or MOU with China.

Israel and China have been close partners in health cooperation. Since the two governments signed the health cooperation agreement in 1993, they have continuously signed health cooperation workplans. The two countries have frequently exchanged high-level health visits since 2011, and steadily forged ahead practical and in-depth cooperation on hospital management, telemedicine, health emergency management, and medical and health technology. China has established good partnership with Afghanistan and Turkey in the health sector, and exchanged ministerial visits with the two countries several times in the area of health. Infectious disease control and prevention is a common area for cooperation. Both countries have planned to set bilateral "Joint Working Commission on Health" with their Chinese counterpart. Saudi Arabia, Iran, and Iraq have limited health cooperation with China, yet China has sent medical experts to these three countries to provide diagnosis and treatment services to their senior officials.

2.5 Central Asia

All of the five Central Asian countries, namely, Kazakhstan, Kyrgyzstan, Tajikistan, Turkmenistan and Uzbekistan, have signed bilateral intergovernmental agreements on health cooperation with China, but actually few health cooperation activities have been carried out between China and these countries. Infectious disease control, prevention, and traditional medicine are commonly emphasized, and due to the difference in national conditions, the areas of cooperation also involve MCH, medical education, health reform, pharmacology, etc. The cooperation between China and Central Asian countries is mainly conducted under the frameworks of the WHO and Shanghai Cooperation Organization.

2.6 Eastern Europe

Russia and Ukraine have established close cooperation partnership with China in the health sector. Both countries have signed bilateral intergovernmental agreement or MOU on health cooperation with China.

In addition to the comprehensive agreement on health cooperation, Russia and China have also signed specific cooperation agreements or MOUs in many areas, such as infectious disease prevention and control, rehabilitation and treatment of children injured in terrorist incidents, and medical treatment as a means of disaster relief. High-level visits are frequently conducted between the two countries in the area of health. Bilateral collaborations have been carried out through various channels, for example, bilateral mechanisms such as the Health Cooperation Sub-Committee of China-Russia Humanities Cooperation Committee, multilateral mechanisms like WHO, Shanghai Cooperation Organization, BRICS and APEC, and collaborations with nongovernmental organizations and institutions. Health cooperation and many medical exchange programs have been robustly advanced between the two countries, including pragmatic activities launched in the fields of traditional medicine, infectious disease control and prevention, and exchanges of professionals and experts among medical institutions.

High-level visits have been conducted several times between Ukraine and China. In the field of health, the two countries have established the Health Cooperation Sub-Committee under the China-Uzbekistan Intergovernmental Cooperation Committee. Meetings are held periodically to promote the cooperation of the two countries in traditional medicine, gerontology, MCH, and medical personnel training.

2.7 North Africa

Egypt and China have signed bilateral intergovernmental MOU on health cooperation, and cooperation needs in the areas of biomedical industry, disease control and prevention, health emergency, population and reproductive health, medical insurance and primary health care have gradually increased.

3 Cholera Risk Assessment, Control, and Prevention

Fengfeng Liu and Biao Kan

Cholera is an acute intestinal infectious disease caused by *Vibrio cholerae* O1 and O139. It is mainly transmitted through *V. cholerae* contaminated water and food. Cholera toxin produced by *V. cholerae* is the main pathogenic factor. The incubation period of cholera is generally several hours to about 5 days. The main clinical symptoms are severe diarrhea and watery stool. Severe cases have complications of severe dehydration and electrolyte disorder [1, 2].

Since 1817, the world has experienced seven cholera pandemics. The seventh pandemic, which began in 1961 and originated in Asia, is still ongoing. The causative pathogen for the seventh pandemic is El Tor biotype *V. cholera* of O1 serogroup [2, 3]. In 1992, a new serogroup—*V. cholerae* O139 that caused cholera was first discovered in India, and now it is mainly prevalent in Asian countries [4].

The study of global cholera disease burden indicates that the estimated annual cholera cases and deaths are 28,600,000 and 95,000, respectively. A total of 69 countries in Sub Saharan Africa and Southeast Asia are cholera endemic countries, accounting for 60% and 29% of global cholera disease burden [5]. In 2018, a total of 499,447 cholera cases and 2990 deaths (CFR = 0.6%) in 34 countries were reported to the WHO [6]. In the cholera endemic countries, the economic burden of cholera is estimated at $2 billion each year, constituted mainly of productivity loss and direct economic loss [7]. As a "poverty disease," the map of cholera prevalence is consistent with the map of extremely poverty areas [7]. Cholera disease control and prevention are one of the most important public health tasks worldwide. In 2017, WHO released "Ending Cholera—A Global Roadmap to 2030," which is

F. Liu
Chinese Center for Disease Control and Prevention, Beijing, People's Republic of China

B. Kan (✉)
National Institute for Communicable Diseases Control and Prevention, China CDC, Beijing, People's Republic of China
e-mail: kanbiao@icdc.cn

W. Yang (ed.), *Prevention and Control of Infectious Diseases in BRI Countries*, https://doi.org/10.1007/978-981-33-6958-0_3

aimed to reduce 90% of cholera deaths globally and eliminate the disease in 20 cholera endemic countries [7].

The risk factors of cholera in "Belt and Road" countries were reviewed in this chapter, including the history and current epidemic, the proportion of the population covered by basic drinking water supply services, sanitation services, hand washing facilities, the disease surveillance system, and the health system. The risk matrix method was applied to assess the level of cholera risk in "Belt and Road" countries by two dimensions, including the probability of the disease occurrence and the consequences of the disease. In order to provide the scientific basis and practical guidance for cholera control in "Belt and Road" countries with cholera outbreaks, containment measures of China were also presented as examples in this chapter.

3.1 The Epidemic Situation of Cholera in "Belt and Road" Countries

The cholera incidence of "Belt and Road" countries was summarized using the Weekly Epidemiological Record (WER) on cholera issued annually by WHO. See Table 3.1 for the data on cases and deaths in "Belt and Road" countries. The countries in which the data were not available from WER were not listed.

3.1.1 Asia Oceania Areas

Malaysia reported a total of 2,983 cholera cases from 2000 to 2017, of which 36 died [8–19]. In Malaysia, the number of reported cholera cases was up to 586, with ten deaths in 2011, but only two cases and no death cases reported in 2017 [10, 14].

Thailand reported a total of 4,701 cholera cases from the year 2006 to 2017, including 33 deaths [9–17, 20–22]. The average annual cases and death were 392 and 3, respectively, over the same period. The number of cases peaked in 2010, with 1,974 cases and 15 deaths [15]. The number of cases was the lowest in 2013 and 2017, with eight cases reported each, and no death [10, 12].

Indonesia reported 1,338 cholera cases in 2005 and 1,007 in 2008, with 19 and 27 deaths, respectively [21, 23].

A total of 7,953 cholera cases were reported in Philippine from 2000 to 2017, of which 41 died [8, 10–15, 17, 18, 22–24]. In 2012 and 2014, the cholera epidemic was serious in Philippine, with 1,864 and 4,547 cases reported, and 14 and 8 deaths, respectively [11, 13]. From 2016 to 2017, the number of cholera cases decreased to over one hundred, and only two deaths were reported [10, 22].

Cambodia reported 57, 39, and 588 cholera cases in 2004, 2009, and 2010, respectively, with two death cases [15, 16, 19].

From 2007 to 2011, the number of cholera cases reported in Vietnam was 1,946, 853, 471, 606, and 3, respectively [14–16, 20, 21]. Only one death was reported over this period [16].

Laos reported 169, 201, and 237 cholera cases, and 3, 0, and 4 deaths, respectively, in 2007, 2008, and 2010 [15, 20, 21].

Table 3.1 Assessed cholera risk levels and number of cholera cases and deaths reported in of "Belt and Road" countries, 2013–2017

	2013[a]		2014[a]		2015[a]		2016[a]		2017[a]		2012–2015[b]		Endemic or not	Assessed Risk level
Country	Cases	Deaths	Cases	Deaths	Cases	Deaths	Cases	Deaths	Cases	Deaths	Cases	Deaths		
Kenya	–	–	35	9	13,291	67	5,866	80	4,288	82	111,273	4,228	+	Very high
Iran	256 (221)*	7	–	–	86 (36)*	1	5	0	634 (625)*	4	–	–	+	Moderate
Iraq	1	0	–	–	4,965	2	3	–	–	–	–	–	+	High
Malaysia	171 (77)*	1	134 (55)*	1	244	2	–	–	2	0	–	–	+	Low
Nepal	–	–	933	2	80	0	169	0	7	0	30,379	911	+	High
Thailand	8	0	12	0	125	1	52	1	8	0	–	–	+	Moderate
Philippines	6	0	4,547	8	–	–	124	0	134	2	2,430	24	+	High
Singapore	2*	0	2*	0	–	–	–	–	3*	0	–	–	–	No
Myanmar	33	0	400	0	103	12	782	11	–	–	–	–	+	High
Russia	–	–	1*	0	–	–	–	–	–	–	–	–	–	No
Israel	1*	0	–	–	–	–	–	–	–	–	–	–	–	No
Vietnam	–	–	–	–	–	–	–	–	–	–	–	–	–	Moderate
Ukraine	–	–	–	–	–	–	–	–	–	–	–	–	–	No
Indonesia	–	–	–	–	–	–	–	–	–	–	2,298	23	+	High
Laos	–	–	–	–	–	–	–	–	–	–	333	3	+	Moderate
Cambodia	–	–	–	–	–	–	–	–	–	–	991	10	+	High
Bangladesh	–	–	–	–	–	–	–	–	–	–	109,052	3,272	+	Very high
Ethiopia	–	–	–	–	–	–	–	–	–	–	275,221	10,458	+	Very high
Uzbekistan	–	–	–	–	–	–	–	–	–	–	–	–	–	Low
Turkmenistan	–	–	–	–	–	–	–	–	–	–	–	–	–	Low
Mongolia	–	–	–	–	–	–	–	–	–	–	–	–	–	Low
Maldives	–	–	–	–	–	–	–	–	–	–	–	–	–	Low
Brunei	–	–	–	–	–	–	–	–	–	–	–	–	–	No

(continued)

Table 3.1 (continued)

	2013[a]		2014[a]		2015[a]		2016[a]		2017[a]		2012–2015[b]		Endemic or not	Assessed Risk level
Country	Cases	Deaths	Cases	Deaths	Cases	Deaths	Cases	Deaths	Cases	Deaths	Cases	Deaths		
Turkey	–	–	–	–	–	–	–	–	–	–	–	–	–	No
Sri Lanka	–	–	–	–	–	–	–	–	–	–	–	–	–	Low
Saudi Arabia	–	–	–	–	–	–	–	–	5*	0	–	–	–	No
Egypt	–	–	–	–	–	–	–	–	–	–	–	–	–	No
Afghanistan	3,957	14	45,481	4	58,064	8	677	5	33	1	29,341	939	+	Very high
India	6,008	54	4,031	21	889	4	841	3	385	3	675,188	20,256	+	Very high
United Arab Emirates	–	–	–	–	–	–	–	–	12*	–	–	–	–	No
Pakistan	1,069	23	1,218	6	–	–	–	–	–	–	–	–	–	High
Tajikistan	–	–	–	–	–	–	–	–	–	–	46	0	+	Moderate
Kyrgyzstan	–	–	–	–	–	–	–	–	–	–	–	–	–	Low
Kazakhstan	–	–	–	–	–	–	–	–	–	–	–	–	–	No

*Imported case; [a]Number of reported cholera cases and deaths from WER published by WHO from 2013 to 2017; [b]Estimated annual number of cholera cases and deaths from cholera disease burden study published by Ali M and others; + Cholera endemic countries; – Cholera none endemic countries. – No data was available from WHO and cholera disease burden study published by Ali M and others

Myanmar reported a total of 1,553 cholera cases, including 24 deaths, in 2008, and from 2011 to 2016 [9, 11–14, 21, 22]. The number of reported cases was relatively high in 2016, with 782 cases and 11 deaths [22].

Singapore reported a total of 18 cholera cases in 2000 and 2001, with no deaths [8, 18]. From 2002 to 2004, 14 cholera cases were reported, of whom two were imported cases and one died [19, 24, 25]. No cholera cases were reported to WHO in years from 2005 to 2010. A total of 11 imported cases were reported from 2011 to 2014 and 2017, no local cases were reported in this period [10–14].

Three imported cases were reported in Brunei in 2011 [14].

3.1.2 Central Asia

Kazakhstan reported one imported cholera case in 2001 and 2008, respectively [8, 21].

3.1.3 Western Asia

A total of 4,203 cholera cases were reported in Iran from 2000 to 2017, of which 44 cases died [8–10, 12–14, 18–25]. The reported number was high in 2005 and 2011, with 1,133, 1,187 cholera cases, and 11, 12 deaths, respectively [14, 23]. After 2012, the number of reported cases decreased significantly in Iran. Only five cases were reported in 2016, but the reported cases increased in 2017, with a total of 634 cases and 4 deaths, among whom 625 were imported cases [10, 22].

A total of 16,763 cholera cases were reported in Iraq from 2000 to 2016, of whom 45 died [9, 12, 13, 15, 16, 18–22, 24, 25]. There were more than 4,000 cases reported in each year of 2007, 2012, and 2015 [9, 13, 20]. Only three cholera cases were reported in 2016 [22].

Three and twelve imported cases were reported in 2002 and 2017, respectively, in the United Arab Emirates [10, 25].

Thirty-eight local cholera cases were reported, with no deaths, in Saudi Arabia in 2002 [25]. There were five imported cases but no deaths in 2017 [10].

Israel reported one imported case in 2013 [12].

Yemen reported 15,751 suspected cholera cases in 2016 [22]. There was a large outbreak in Yemen in 2017, with a total of 1,032,481 suspected cases and 2,261 deaths reported, making it the only country with more than one million cases reported in a year [10]. In 2018, it reported 371,326 cases and 505 deaths [6].

3.1.4 South Asia

The cholera epidemic was serious in Afghanistan. From 2000 to 2017, a total of 128,278 cholera cases were reported, in whom 438 died [8–16, 18, 21–25]. The number peaked in 2014 and 2015, or 45,481 and 58,064, respectively [9, 11]. The epidemic took a turn for the better in 2016 and 2017, with 677 and 33 cases reported, 5 and 1 death, respectively [10, 22].

A total of 3,122 cholera cases were reported in Pakistan between 2010 and 2014, including 256 deaths [11–15]; 527 cholera cases and 219 deaths were reported in 2011, and the case fatality rate, 42% [14]. The epidemics of cholera were still serious in Pakistan from 2013 to 2014, with 1,069 and 1,218 cases reported, respectively. The reported number of deaths was 29 in this period of time [11, 12].

A total of 46,649 cholera cases were reported in India from 2000 to 2017, including 150 deaths [8–12, 15, 17–25]. From 2000 to 2014, the annual average of cholera cases and deaths were 3,711 and 12, respectively [8, 11, 12, 15, 17–21, 23–25]. The number of reported cases decreased significantly from 2015 to 2017, with an average of 705 cases and three deaths reported [9, 10, 22].

Sri Lanka only reported cholera cases to WHO in 2000 and 2002. A total of 11 cholera cases and 1 death was reported [18, 25].

A total of 3,371 cholera cases were reported in Nepal from 2007 to 2017, including 11 deaths [9–11, 13–16, 20, 22]. The peak appeared in 2010, with 1,790 cases and nine deaths reported [15]. The number of cases bottomed out in 2017, with seven cases and no death [10]. From 2007 to 2017, the yearly average of reported case and death was 375 and 1, respectively.

3.1.5 Eastern Europe

Fifty-three cholera cases were reported in Russia in 2001 without mortality [8]. There was one imported case in each year of 2004, 2006, 2012, and 2014 [11, 13, 19, 20]. Three imported cases were reported in 2010 [15].

Ukraine reported one imported case in 2007 and 33 local cases in 2011, with no deaths [14, 20].

3.1.6 Africa

The cholera epidemic was very serious in the history of Ethiopia. A total of 115,260 cholera cases were reported between 2004 and 2010, including 1,325 deaths [15–17, 19–21]. No cholera cases were reported to WHO from 2011 to 2017. However, in the study of the global burden of cholera published by Ali M and others in 2015, the cholera cases and death in Ethiopia were estimated at 275,221 and 10,458, respectively, hence the fatality rate, 3.8% [5].

The cholera epidemic was serious in Kenya. A total of 47,469 cholera cases were reported from 2000 to 2017, including 937 deaths [8–11, 14–23, 25]. Tens of thousands of cholera cases were reported in 2009 and 2015 [9, 16]. From 2015 to 2017, the yearly average of reported cases and deaths were 7,815 and 76, respectively.

3.2 The Cholera Risk Level in "Belt and Road" Countries and the Principles for Cholera Control

3.2.1 Principles and Basis for the Assessment of Cholera Risk Level

1. The risk matrix method [26] was applied to assess the level of cholera risk in "Belt and Road" countries by two dimensions, including the probability of the disease occurrence and the consequences of the disease.
2. According to the number of cholera cases and deaths reported by WHO from 2000 to 2017, the probability of cholera occurrence in different countries was assessed. In view of the defective surveillance system, inconsistent case definition, lack of laboratory diagnostic capacity, and the impact on trade and tourism, it is estimated that only 5–10% of cholera cases are reported to WHO every year [5, 27, 28]. Therefore, the results from the study of the updated global burden of cholera in endemic countries conducted by Ali M and others were used to correct the number of reported cases from WHO in each country.
3. The indicators of the proportion of the population covered by basic drinking water services, sanitation services, and handwashing facilities released by WHO in 2015 were used to assess the probability of cholera occurrence and risk level in "Belt and Road" countries. See Table 3.2 for the coverage of basic drinking water services, sanitation services, and handwashing facilities in "Belt and Road" countries.
4. In addition to the incidence and occurrence risk factors of cholera, other risk factors such as medical and health level, political environment, infectious disease surveillance system, etc., of each country were also referred to when correcting the assessed risk level of cholera.

3.2.2 Assessed Cholera Risk Level of "Belt and Road" Countries

3.2.2.1 Countries with Very High Risk of Cholera

3.2.2.1.1 Ethiopia, Kenya

It was estimated that more than 100,000 cholera cases and 10,000 deaths occur annually in Ethiopia and Kenya, respectively [5]. In 2015, the proportion of population covered by basic drinking water services in Ethiopia and Kenya was low, 39% and 58%, respectively, and the proportion of people using untreated surface water sources was high, or 12% and 23%, respectively [29]. The water supply facilities of the two countries were backward, and the proportion of population covered by pipeline water supply was approximately 30% [29]. Sanitation facilities were seriously outdated in Ethiopia and Kenya, and the coverage, 7% and 30%, respectively [29]. In Ethiopia, the percentage of open defecation was 27% [29]. The coverage of

Table 3.2 The proportion of population covered by drinking water, sanitation, and hand washing facilities of "Belt and Road" countries, 2015

Country	Proportion of population covered by basic drinking water services (%)	Proportion of population covered by basic sanitation services (%)	Proportion of population covered by hand washing facility (%)
Ethiopia	39	7	1
Kenya	58	30	14
Afghanistan	63	39	38
Myanmar	68	65	80
Tajikistan	74	95	73
Cambodia	75	49	66
Laos	80	73	–
Mongolia	83	59	72
Iraq	86	86	91
Kyrgyzstan	87	97	89
Pakistan	89	58	60
Nepal	88	46	57
India	88	44	–
Indonesia	90	68	77
Philippines	91	75	–
Vietnam	91	78	86
Kazakhstan	91	98	96
Sri Lanka	92	94	–
Turkmenistan	94	97	98
Iran	95	88	–
Malaysia	96	100	–
Russia	96	89	–
Bangladesh	97	47	40
Thailand	98	95	–
Ukraine	98	96	–
Maldives	98	96	–
Egypt	98	93	88
Turkey	99	96	–
Singapore	100	100	–
Israel	100	100	–
Brunei	100	96	–
Saudi Arabia	100	100	–
United Arab Emirates	100	100	–
Uzbekistan[a]	99	100	–

[a]Urban areas; – Data not available

handwashing facilities in both countries was also low, that is, 1% in Ethiopia and 14% in Kenya [29].

In terms of the medical and health system and infectious disease surveillance system, both countries are short of health human resources. Ethiopia has infectious disease surveillance system but lacks the literature for effect evaluation. The infectious disease surveillance system in Kenya is backward, and its infectious disease reporting is based on text message [30].

3.2.2.1.2 Bangladesh

There is no national cholera surveillance system with laboratory diagnosis in Bangladesh, and no epidemic of cholera is reported officially. The Bangladesh Institute for Epidemiological Disease Control estimates that the annual number of cholera cases in Bangladesh is 450,000 [31]. The International Research Center for Diarrhoeal Diseases in Bangladesh estimates that a total of 300,000 severe cholera cases needed to be hospitalized in the country every year [31]. According to the study of global cholera burden of endemic countries, the estimated annual number of its cholera cases and deaths is 109,052 and 3,272, respectively [5]. Thanks to the urban pipeline water supply construction and water treatment facilities project, the coverage of basic drinking water services reached 97% in 2015, but of advanced water supply facilities at safety management level, only 56% [29, 31]. The coverage of handwashing facilities was 40%, which was quite low [29]. Only half of the population receive basic sanitation services, and the sanitation facilities of 31% of the population were backward [29]. In addition, Bangladesh is the least developed country, lacking both medical personnel and medical supplies [30].

3.2.2.1.3 Afghanistan

The epidemic of cholera disease is very serious in Afghanistan. Although only 33 cholera cases were reported to WHO in 2017, it is estimated that the actual annual number is about 30,000, and the deaths, nearly 1,000 [5, 10]. Years of war have caused serious damage to water supply, health infrastructure, and healthcare system in Afghanistan. In 2015, the proportion of the population covered by basic drinking water services was 63%, by pipeline water supply, only 12%, and the proportion of population using untreated surface water sources, 15% [29]. The coverage of handwashing facilities was only 38% [29]. Sanitation facilities were seriously backward in Afghanistan, and only 39% of the population was covered by basic sanitation services in 2015 [29]. The proportion of open defecation in rural areas was 18%, and only 3% of the population benefitted from the improved sanitation facility of sewer connections in 2015 in Afghanistan [29].

3.2.2.1.4 India

Cholera epidemic is an important public health challenge to India. Studies estimated that the annual number of cholera cases in India is 675,188, with 20,256 deaths [5]. In 2015, the proportion of the population covered by basic drinking water services was 88%, and that of those using pipeline water and untreated surface water was 43% and 1%, respectively [29]. The proportion of the population covered by basic sanitation services and sewer connections was 44% and 9%, respectively, in 2015 [29]. The proportion of open defecation was as high as 40% in the same year [29]. In 2014, India implemented the national sanitation program Swachh Bharat Mission (SBM), which was designed to eliminate open defecation in 2019. According to SBM data, the coverage of latrines in rural areas was 65% in 2017, and the number of people practicing open defecation declined from 550 million to 330 million [29]. Although cholera is one of the 18 notifiable infectious diseases in India, the corresponding surveillance system is defective, and there is always a failure to report [32]. Despite the adoption of some control measures, including improving sanitation facilities and quitting habits of open defecation, the shortage of cholera vaccines and the extensive exposure to the disease have made it a big threat to India.

3.2.2.2 Countries with a High Risk of Cholera

3.2.2.2.1 Pakistan

No cholera cases were reported by Pakistan to WHO between 2015 and 2017. However, the number of cholera cases was relatively high from 2013 to 2014 when more than one thousand cases were reported in Pakistan [11, 12]. According to the global cholera disease burden study conducted by Ali M and others, Pakistan was a nonendemic country, which indicated that the burden of cholera might be different by region in Pakistan [5]. The surveillance system in Pakistan includes the response monitoring of outbreaks of acute watery diarrhea/suspected cholera, Disease Early Warning System (DEWS), and Integrated Disease Surveillance and Response System (IDSRS), all being linked with a public health laboratory in provinces of Punjab and Sindh [33].

From 2011 to 2014, DEWS reported over one million cases of acute watery diarrhea, of which 787 were acute watery diarrhea or suspected cholera outbreaks [33]. From 2013 to 2016, nonaggregated data of Punjab indicated that 8.9% of acute watery diarrhea cases were suspected cholera cases [33]. A total of 2,958 cholera cases were reported between 2011 and 2015 by WHO, with the average number of cholera cases, 592. In 2015, the proportion of population covered by basic drinking water services, pipeline water supply, and of people using untreated surface water sources was 89%, 33%, and 2%, respectively, in Pakistan [29]. The sanitation facilities was backward, and only 58% of the population covered by basic sanitation services [29]. There was still 12% of the population practicing open defecation in 2015, and 60% of the population had access to handwashing facilities [29].

Although Pakistan has relatively completed disease surveillance systems, the detection rate of *V. cholerae* culture is low. In addition, risk factors such as the increasing density of urban population and climate changes caused by aggravated environmental pollution have further increased the risk of cholera in Pakistan [34].

3.2.2.2.2 Nepal

The epidemic situation of cholera in Nepal was very serious in history. A total of 92,000 cholera cases and 1,800 deaths were reported in 1991 [31]. Though no cholera cases were reported to WHO between 2000 and 2006. From 2007 to 2014, there was an average number of 519 cases and two deaths were reported to WHO [11,

13–16, 20]. In recent years, the reported cases decreased later, that is, 80, 169, and 7 in 2015, 2016, and 2017, respectively [9, 10, 22]. In 2015, the population covered by basic drinking water services, basic sanitation services, hand washing facilities accounted for 88%, 46%, and 57%, respectively [29]. The proportion of people practicing open defecation was up to 30% in 2015 [29]. Although the reported number of cholera cases to WHO has declined in recent years, the annual cholera cases and deaths were estimated at 30, 379, and 911, respectively [5]. The economy is backward in Nepal, and its health care personnel and health resources are limited, which also increase the risk of cholera in Nepal.

3.2.2.2.3 Iraq

Only three cases were reported to WHO in 2016 from Iraq [22]. However, more than 4,000 cases were reported to WHO in 2015, including 2,800 cases and two deaths from an outbreak downstream of the Euphrates River and due to the destruction of water supply facilities [9, 35]. The proportion of people covered by basic drinking water services and of those using untreated surface water sources was 86% and 3% in 2015 [29]. The coverage of pipeline water supply in rural and urban areas was unbalanced, or 90% and 65%, respectively [29]. The proportion of the population covered by basic sanitation services was 86%, and sanitation facilities for 4% of the population were still backward in 2015 [29]. The coverage of handwashing facilities was 91% that year [29].

After the war, the recovery of Iraq's public health system was slow, the medical and health system suffered major damages, and the coverage of safe drinking water was unbalanced [36]. Once a local conflict should occur, cholera could easily spread in local areas, hence a high risk of cholera in the country.

3.2.2.2.4 Indonesia

No cholera data of Indonesia were found in WER published by WHO from 2000 to 2017. It is estimated that its annual cholera cases and deaths are 2,298 and 23, respectively [5]. In 2015, the proportion of the population covered by basic drinking water services, pipeline water supply, basic sanitation services, and handwashing facilities was 90%, 18%, 68%, and 77%, respectively [29]. Twelve percent of the population practiced open defecation in 2015 [29]. The public health system was backward, the medical resources were limited [30], hence high risk of cholera in Indonesia.

3.2.2.2.5 Philippines

In the Philippines, the estimated annual number of cholera cases and deaths was 2,430 and 24, respectively [5]. The population coverage of basic drinking water services and of the supply of pipelines was 91% and 43%, respectively, in 2015 [29]. However, the sanitation facilities were backward, the population coverage of basic sanitation services was 75%, and 6% of its people practiced open defecation in 2015 [29]. From 2011 to 2016, the event-based outbreak and response monitoring system reported a total of 66 cholera outbreaks in the Philippines, when the death cases totaled 156 [33]. In 2016, 30 cholera outbreaks and 22 deaths were reported [33], indicating a high risk of cholera in the Philippines.

3.2.2.2.6 Myanmar

A total of 1,508 cholera cases and 23 deaths were reported in Myanmar from 2011 to 2016, with an annual average of 251 cases and 4 deaths [9, 11–14, 22]. Seven-hundred and eighty-two cholera cases and eleven deaths were reported in 2016 [22]. There were insufficient drinking water and sanitation facilities in Myanmar, covering 68% and 65% of the population, respectively, in 2015 [29]. Five percent of the population practiced open defecation and the population coverage of handwashing facilities was 80% in 2015 [29]. Therefore, the cholera risk is high in Myanmar.

3.2.2.2.7 Cambodia

No confirmed cholera cases were reported in Cambodia from 2011 to 2015, but the number of acute watery diarrhea was 287,330–363,078 between 2011 and 2015 [33]. Ali M and others estimated that the annual number of cholera and deaths was 991 and 10 in Cambodia [5]. The population coverage of basic drinking water services, basic sanitation services, and handwashing facilities was 75%, 49%, and 66%, respectively, in 2015 [29]. The proportion of population practicing open defecation was up to 41% the same year [29]. Therefore, the risk of cholera is high in Cambodia.

3.2.2.3 Countries with a Moderate Risk of Cholera

3.2.2.3.1 Iran

Iran is a cholera endemic country, but the number of reported cholera cases has declined in recent years. There were 86 (36 imported cases), 5, and 634 cases (625 imported cases) reported in 2015, 2016, and 2017, respectively, and a total of five deaths during this period of time [9, 10, 22]. In Iran, the population coverage of basic drinking water services, pipeline water supply, basic sanitation services was relatively high, or 95%, 93%, and 88%, respectively, in 2015 [29]. The proportion of population practicing open defecation and of that using outdated sanitation facilities was both 1% in 2015 [29]. There is a complete healthcare system in Iran. Despite the infectious disease surveillance system it has, the absence of a unified disease reporting information system leads to a low disease reporting rate [30]. The delay in reporting inevitably makes cholera outbreak and spread possible; therefore, the level of cholera risk is moderate in Iran.

3.2.2.3.2 Laos

The annual number of cholera cases and deaths is estimated at 333 and 3, respectively, in Laos [5]. The population coverage of basic drinking water services, pipeline water supply, and basic sanitation services was 80%, 42% and 73%, respectively, in 2015 [29]. There were 22% of the population practicing open defecation [29]. The level of cholera risk is moderate in Laos.

3.2.2.3.3 Vietnam

Although no cholera cases had been reported in Vietnam since 2012, there were hundreds of thousands of acute watery diarrhea cases reported from 2011 to 2015 [33]. The population coverage of basic drinking water services and handwashing facilities was 91% and 86%, respectively, in 2015, but of basic sanitation services, relatively low, or 78% [29]. The report of cholera is statutory in Vietnam. The country has national disease surveillance for acute watery diarrhea and suspected surveillance system, and its provincial medical institutions have the ability to detect cholera. The suspected cholera outbreaks are reported to local public health departments through special lines [33]. Therefore, the level of cholera risk is moderate in Vietnam.

3.2.2.3.4 Thailand

The average number of cholera cases and deaths was 392 and 3, respectively, in Thailand from 2006 to 2017, but in recent years, the number has declined. In 2017, only eight cases were reported, with no death [10]. Its population coverage of basic drinking water services and basic sanitation services was high in 2015, 98% and 95%, respectively [29]. The report of cholera is statutory in Thailand [33]. It has an event-based monitoring system for acute diarrhea and food poisoning [33]. Provincial and large regional hospitals have the ability to culture and detect *V. cholerae* [33].

3.2.2.4 Countries with Low Risk of Cholera

3.2.2.4.1 Malaysia

There has been no cholera epidemic in most parts of Malaysia, and 90% of cholera cases are mainly concentrated in Sabah [33]. The average number of cholera cases was 264 in Malaysia from 2011 to 2015. The incidence of cholera has dropped from 1.8 per 100,000 people in 2011 to 0.5 per 100,000 in 2016 [33]. The report of cholera is statutory in Malaysia. Cholera monitoring surveillance was established in 1988 [33]. Once identified as a suspected case, the person will be required to report to the public health department within 24 h [33]. All suspected cases are tested by means of a bacterial culture [33]. Confirmed cases are registered on the e-notice network platform [33]. Its population coverage of basic drinking water services, pipeline water supply, and basic sanitation services was 92%, 94%, and 100%, respectively, in 2015 [29].

3.2.2.4.2 Mongolia

In 1996, there was a cholera outbreak in Mongolia, when more than 100 cases and eight deaths were reported [37]. No cholera cases have been reported in recent years. The public health construction is backward, and the government does not attach great importance to disease prevention in Mongolia [30]. The population coverage of basic drinking water services, basic sanitation services, and handwashing facilities was 83%, 59%, and 72%, respectively, in 2015 [29]. The proportion of people using a surface water source was 5%, and the proportion practicing open defecation, 10% [29]. Therefore, the probability of cholera occurrence is not excluded in Mongolia, despite the low risk.

3.2.2.4.3 Maldives

In the Maldives, the population coverage of basic drinking water services and basic sanitation services were both over 95%, but the coverage of water supply facilities was unbalanced [29]. There was no pipeline water supply in rural areas, and the sanitation facilities in rural areas were relatively backward. The coverage of sewer connections in rural areas was 22% [29]. In addition, Maldives is geographically adjacent to India, where the cholera epidemic is serious. Although no cholera cases were reported from the Maldives and the risk is low, the probability of cholera occurrence still exists.

3.2.2.4.4 Uzbekistan

A cholera outbreak was reported in 1990 in Samarkand Province of Uzbekistan [38]. No cholera cases have been reported in recent years in Uzbekistan. The public health system is not complete, and the burden of intestinal infectious diseases is heavy in Uzbekistan [30]. Although the population coverage of basic drinking water services in urban areas and the basic sanitation services was 99% and 100%, respectively, in 2015, the interruption of water supply and the pollution of water sources were among the main problems Uzbekistan encounters [29, 30]. There is no report of cholera epidemic in Uzbekistan, but the drinking water is not safe, the sanitation facilities are backward, the environment is seriously polluted, and the incidence of intestinal infectious diseases is high, so the probability of cholera occurrence is not excluded in Uzbekistan.

3.2.2.4.5 Sri Lanka

An El Tor cholera outbreak was reported from Sri Lanka in the 1970s [31]. A total of eleven cholera cases and one death were reported to the WHO between 2000 and 2002 [18, 25]. The population coverage of basic drinking water services was 92%; however, the water supply facilities were backward, and only 38% of the population was covered by pipeline water supply in 2015 [29]. The population coverage of basic sanitation facilities was 94%, and of the population practicing open defecation, 3% in 2015 [29]. In 2016, the mortality rate due to unsafe water, unsafe sanitation, and lack of hygiene was 1.2 per 100,000 people in Sri Lanka [39]. The risk of cholera is low in Sri Lanka.

3.2.2.5 Cholera Risk Level in Central Asian Countries

In central Asian countries, except for an annual number of 46 cholera cases in Tajikistan as was estimated by Ali M and others, and imported cholera cases reported in Kazakhstan, no cholera data of other countries was found [5, 8, 21]. The population coverage of the basic drinking water services, basic sanitation services, and handwashing facilities was 74%, 95%, and 73%, respectively, in 2015 in Tajikistan [29]. Therefore, the risk level of cholera is moderate in Tajikistan. Kazakhstan is not a cholera endemic country [30]. The population coverage of basic drinking water services and basic sanitation services was both over 90% in 2015 [29]. Therefore, there is no risk of cholera in Kazakhstan. In Turkmenistan, the mortality rate due to unsafe water, unsafe sanitation, and lack of hygiene was 4.0 per 100,000 people, and the government banned reporting cholera, tuberculosis, and other infectious diseases in 2004, which furthered the spread of infectious diseases [30, 39]. Therefore, the probability of cholera occurrence in Turkmenistan cannot be excluded. In 2015, its population coverage of basic drinking water services, pipeline water supply, basic sanitation services, hand washing facilities was 87%, 89%, 97%, 89%, respectively [29], indicating a low risk level of cholera in Kyrgyzstan.

3.2.2.6 Countries Without Cholera Risk

Singapore, Russia, Ukraine, Egypt, Israel, Saudi Arabia, the United Arab Emirates, Turkey, and Brunei are cholera nonendemic countries. Between 2013 and 2017, except for the United Arab Emirates, Russia, Singapore, Israel, and Saudi Arabia, no imported cases were reported in other countries, and the drinking water is safe and the sanitation facilities are improved.

3.2.3 General Principles for Cholera Prevention and Control

The general principles for cholera prevention and control are to provide safe drinking water, improve sanitation facilities and personal hygiene, provide timely treatment, conduct health education, enhance community engagement, and expand cholera vaccination [7, 40, 41].

Cholera vaccine is an effective prevention and control measure to control the cholera outbreak and epidemic. WHO recommends the cholera vaccines should be a top choice in areas with a high risk of cholera endemic, as well as in humanitarian crises with a high risk of cholera. The use of vaccine must be combined with other cholera prevention and control measures, and should not hinder the adoption of other health interventions. When the resources are limited, the high-risk groups, such as infants of 1-year-old and above and pregnant women, should be immunized first [42].

In 2017, WHO launched the "Ending Cholera—A Global Roadmap to 2030" that included three cholera prevention and control strategies [7]. First, early detection and quick response to contain outbreaks, such as by strengthening community engagement, early warning surveillance, laboratory testing capacity, health systems and supply readiness, and establishing rapid emergency response teams. Second, develop a targeted multisectoral approach to prevent cholera recurrence and focus on areas of high incidence of cholera (areas that usually have seasonal epidemics, or that play an important role in the spread of cholera). The main measures of cholera prevention and control in hotspots areas are to provide safe drinking water, ensure adequate sanitation facilities, improve personal hygiene, wash hands, and apply cholera vaccine. Third, an effective mechanism of coordination for technical support, advocacy, resource mobilization, and partnership at local and global levels. The Global Task Force on Cholera Control (GTFCC) of WHO has established a strong cooperation mechanism to support cholera control in countries and will provide human, technical, and financial support [7].

Prevention and Control of Cholera—Cases

Fujian is located in the southeast of China, and it is the start of Maritime Silk Road. The cholera outbreak in 2005 in Fujian is the biggest one after year 2000 in China. In the response to this cholera outbreak, both advanced molecular technique and traditional epidemiology investigation were involved. Every single cholera case was investigated and each *Vibrio cholerae* strain was analyzed in the lab. In response to this cholera outbreak, government management and administrative support are the basis, scientific decision-making, precise containment measure, and economic supports are the key points.

1. Response to a Cholera Outbreak in Fujian, China in 2005

In 2005, a total of 205 confirmed cholera cases and 6 carriers were reported in Fuzhou and 10 counties (cities) were affected. The first case was reported in Jinan District, Fuzhou City on August 12, 2005. The numbers of newly reported cases peaked between September 5 and September 13, but decreased significantly in late September. The last case was reported on October 5. The majority of cholera cases were young adults, with 59.5% aged from 20 to 49. Different from previous epidemics, most of the cholera cases (66.8%) in Fuzhou in 2005 reported were from urban areas. In previous epidemics, the cases reported were mainly from coastal suburban counties. Among these 211 cases, 208 were infected with serogroup O1 El Tor *V. cholerae* and the serotype was Inaba. One case was infected with serogroup O1 El Tor Ogawa *V. cholerae*, and the remaining two cases were infected with Serogroup O139 *V. cholerae*.

As soon as the first cholera case was found, Fuzhou CDC directly reported the case to China CDC through the National Internet-Based Infectious Diseases Reporting System and carried out epidemiological investigation and laboratory analysis simultaneously. In September, cholera cases continued to appear in urban areas and suburban counties of Fuzhou. Therefore, the Ministry of Health and Fujian Health Administrative Department dispatched national and provincial experts to Fuzhou. There they worked together with local disease control and prevention staff. The main measures included the following: (1) The establishment of a comprehensive coordination and management mechanism under the guidance of Fuzhou Municipal Government, the leadership of Fuzhou Municipal Health Bureau, together with other administrative departments in Fuzhou; (2) public health education on diarrheal diseases, and enhanced management of drinking water, food, restaurants, and mobile vendors led by the public health administrative department of Fuzhou Municipal Government; (3) enhanced management and treatment of patients, suspected cases, close contacts to patient's excreta; (4) active monitoring, including isolation and identification of *V. cholerae* in vulnerable population, suspicious food and environmental water samples, active surveillance of patients and carriers, determination of infection factor; (5) pulsed field gel electrophoresis (PFGE) molecular subtyping analysis on *V. cholerae* strains isolated from patients, analysis of environmental and food samples for source tracking and risk assessment.

In the response to the cholera outbreak in Fuzhou in 2005, the establishment of a comprehensive coordination and investigation mechanism guided by the government, led by the health administration department, and that involved relevant departments is an important factor to ensure the investigation of and response to the cholera outbreak. Improving the public awareness of preventing infectious diseases through extensive health education played an important role in response to the diseases. Laboratory testing and surveillance based on the molecular typing technique of *V. cholerae* provided critical evidence for identifying outbreak sources and transmission routes. The combination of laboratory analysis and epidemiological investigations provided an essential assurance for the control of cholera outbreak.

2. Containment Strategies of O139 Cholerae in South of Xinjiang in 1993, China

In 1992, *V. cholerae* O139, a new serogroup of *V. cholerae* caused the outbreak and prevalence of cholera in South Asia and attracted worldwide attention. In late May 1993, the first case of *V. cholerae* O139 in China occurred in Keping County, Aksu district, Xinjiang. By the middle of September, a total of 200 cholera cases, 4 deaths, and 225 carriers were reported. The cholera cases were distributed in five counties of Kashgar and Aksu regions. To be specific, 165 cholera cases were found in the Keping County, with an incidence rate of 448.5 per 100,000, which indicated an outbreak, and only sporadic cases were found in the other four counties. That was the first cholera outbreak caused by *V. cholerae* O139 in China. It lasted for a long time (115 days) and spread widely (thirteen towns and villages in five counties in two regions). The strains were multiple-drug resistant (common antibiotics, including compound sulfamethoxazole, streptomycin, and furazolidone), which made the treatment very difficult, prolonged the disease course, and lead to many severe cases.

In the early stage of the epidemic, the Chinese government and CDC staffs carried out a systematic epidemiological investigation and laboratory testing analysis. First, they carried out laboratory test in time to determine the serogroup of *V. cholerae* O139, which provided a scientific basis for prevention and control measures. One and a half months after *V. cholerae* O139 was first detected, the first batch of high titer diagnostic serum was developed and produced for rapid diagnosis of subsequent cases. Second, they performed active surveillance, detected *V. cholerae* for suspected populations and environment, including close contacts, people in epidemic areas, entry-exit persons, and water samples from the environment. In the first 10 days of July, two carriers infected by O139 serogroup were detected in the lafu of Hongqi Port, and after then, the detection and management of the entry personnel were strengthened. Third, the infection routes were analyzed through the epidemiological investigation of early cases. The results indicated that the epidemic was mainly caused by contaminated water and food. Based on the above findings, the Chinese government and health administrative departments strengthened the administrative intervention measures, and urged the implementation of disease prevention measures. The "One Publicity, Four Management Activities and One Big Health Campaign" strategy was launched, namely, to strengthen the propagation on disease prevention, to conscientiously manage water, feces, food and patients, and to conduct a mass patriotic health campaign. In 1994, no outbreak caused by O139 was reported in local areas, and the molecular subtype of O139 isolated from sporadic cases in other provinces of China was quite different from that of Xinjiang found in 1993. This indicated that the epidemic of cholera in southern Xinjiang was successfully controlled and did not continue in local areas or spread to other areas of China.

In the prevention and control of cholera outbreaks or epidemics, government management and administrative support are the basis; scientific decision-making and precise containment measures are the key points. In the early stage of cholera epidemic, the key measure of identifying and controlling the spread of the disease was to determine the serogroup of epidemic causative strains and establish a rapid and effective detection method. Meanwhile, active surveillance should be carried out to strengthen the detection and management of the key population. The epidemiological investigation should be carried out as soon as possible, and the infection routes should be analyzed, so as to provide a scientific basis for the formulation of prevention and control measures.

References

1. Donglou X. Cholera Control Handbook (6th edition). Beijing, China: People's Medical Publishing House; 2013.
2. Clemens JD, Nair GB, Ahmed T, Qadri F, Holmgren J. Cholera. Lancet (London, England). 2017;390(10101):1539–49.
3. Deen J, Mengel MA, Clemens JD. Epidemiology of cholera. Vaccine. 2019;38:A31–40.
4. Murugaiah C. The burden of cholera. Crit Rev Microbiol. 2011;37(4):337–48.

5. Ali M, Lopez AL, You YA, et al. The global burden of cholera. Bull World Health Organ. 2012;90(3):209–18A.
6. World Health Organization. Cholera, 2018. Wkly Epidemiol Rec. 2019;94(48):561–8.
7. WHO. Ending cholera A global roadmap to 2030. Geneva: WHO; 2017.
8. World Health Organization. Cholera, 2001. Wkly Epidemiol Rec. 2002;77(31):257–68.
9. World Health Organization. Cholera, 2015. Wkly Epidemiol Rec. 2016;91(38):433–40.
10. World Health Organization. Cholera, 2017. Wkly Epidemiol Rec. 2018;93(38):489–500.
11. World Health Organization. Cholera, 2014. Wkly Epidemiol Rec. 2015;90(40):517–44.
12. World Health Organization. Cholera, 2013. Wkly Epidemiol Rec. 2014;89(31):345–56.
13. World Health Organization. Cholera, 2012. Wkly Epidemiol Rec. 2013;88(31):321–36.
14. World Health Organization. Cholera, 2011. Wkly Epidemiol Rec. 2012;87(31–32):289–304.
15. World Health Organization. Cholera, 2010. Wkly Epidemiol Rec. 2011;86(31):325–40.
16. World Health Organization. Cholera, 2009. Wkly Epidemiol Rec. 2010;85(31):293–308.
17. World Health Organization. Cholera, 2006. Wkly Epidemiol Rec. 2007;82(31):273–84.
18. World Health Organization. Cholera, 2000. Wkly Epidemiol Rec. 2001;76(31):233–40.
19. World Health Organization. Cholera, 2004. Wkly Epidemiol Rec. 2005;80(31):261–8.
20. World Health Organization. Cholera, 2007. Wkly Epidemiol Rec. 2008;83(31):261–84.
21. World Health Organization. Cholera, 2008. Wkly Epidemiol Rec. 2009;84(31):309–24.
22. World Health Organization. Cholera, 2016. Wkly Epidemiol Rec. 2017;92(36):521–36.
23. World Health Organization. Cholera, 2005. Wkly Epidemiol Rec. 2006;81(31):297–308.
24. World Health Organization. Cholera, 2003. Wkly Epidemiol Rec. 2004;79(31):281–8.
25. World Health Organization. Cholera, 2002. Wkly Epidemiol Rec. 2003;78(31):269–76.
26. Rapid risk assessment of acute public health events.
27. Mengel MA, Delrieu I, Heyerdahl L, Gessner BD. Cholera outbreaks in Africa. Curr Top Microbiol Immunol. 2014;379:117–44.
28. World Health Statistics. 2018: monitoring health for the SDGs, sustainable development goals. Geneva: World Health Organization; 2018. Licence: CC BY-NC-SA 3.0 IGO.
29. WHO. Progress on drinking water, sanitation and hygiene: 2017 update and SDG baselines. Geneva: World Health Organization (WHO) and the United Nations Children's Fund (UNICEF); 2017. Licence: CC BY-NC-SA 3.0 IGO.
30. Weizhong Y. Risk assessment of infectious diseases for countries along the Belt and Road and suggestions. Beijing, China: People's Medical Publishing House; 2019.
31. Bharati K, Bhattacharya SK. Cholera outbreaks in South-East Asia. Curr Top Microbiol Immunol. 2014;379:87–116.
32. Gupta SS, Ganguly NK. Opportunities and challenges for cholera control in India. Vaccine. 2019;38:A25–7.
33. Lopez AL, Dutta S, Qadri F, et al. Cholera in selected countries in Asia. Vaccine. 2019;38:A18–24.
34. Naseer M, Jamali T. Epidemiology, determinants and dynamics of cholera in Pakistan: gaps and prospects for future research. J College Phys Surg Pak. 2014;24(11):855–60.
35. Bagcchi S. Cholera in Iraq strains the fragile state. Lancet Infect Dis. 2016;16(1):24–5.
36. Devi S. Reconstructing Iraq. Lancet (London, England). 2018;392(10147):541–2.
37. WHO Emergencies preparedness, response1996 Cholerain Mongolia Update 2.
38. Mukhamedov SM, Inzhevatova MV, Seredin VG, Inogamova IA. An outbreak of cholera (El Tor) in Samarkand Province, Uzbekistan in 1990. Zh Mikrobiol Epidemiol Immunobiol. 1992;9–10:34–7.
39. Mortality rate attributed to unsafe water, unsafe sanitation and lack of hygiene WHO 2016; https://apps.who.int/gho/data/node.main.INADEQUATEWSH?lang=en.
40. World Health Organization. Cholera prevention and Control. https://www.who.int/health-topics/cholera#tab=tab_2.
41. Prevention and control of cholera outbreaks: WHO policy and recommendations. https://www.who.int/cholera/prevention_control/recommendations/en/index1.html.
42. Cholera Vaccines. WHO position paper—August 2017. Wkly Epidemiol Rec. 2017;92(34):477–500.

Risk Assessment and Control on Vaccine-Preventable Diseases

4

Qiru Su, Guijun Ning, and Huiming Luo

4.1 Poliomyelitis

Poliomyelitis (polio) is a highly infectious intestinal disease caused by the poliovirus. Poliovirus is transmitted by person-to-person spread mainly through the fecal–oral route, or, less frequently, by contaminated water or food. Humans are the only known reservoir of poliovirus, which is transmitted most frequently by persons with inapparent infections. Initial symptoms of polio include fever, fatigue, headache, vomiting, stiffness in the neck, and pain in the limbs. In a small proportion of cases (1 in 200 infections), poliovirus causes paralysis, which is often permanent. Instead of a cure for polio, it can only be prevented. The Polio vaccines, given multiple times, can protect a child for life.

4.1.1 Overview of Polio in the "Belt and Road" Countries

Wild poliovirus cases have decreased by over 99% since 1988, from an estimated 350,000 cases in more than 125 endemic countries then to 33 reported cases in 2018. There are three individual and immunologically distinct wild poliovirus strains: wild poliovirus type 1 (WPV1), wild poliovirus type 2 (WPV2), and wild poliovirus type 3 (WPV3). WPV3 and WPV2 were announced, by WHO, to be eradicated in 2015 and 2019, respectively. The last case of WPV3 was detected in Northern Nigeria in 2012 [1]. Eighty-eight confirmed WPV1 cases were reported from January 1 to October 15, 2019, including 72 in Pakistan and 16 in Afghanistan, 3.4 times more than that of the same period (20) in 2018, and also more than the

Q. Su · G. Ning · H. Luo (✉)
Chinese Center for Disease Control and Prevention, Beijing, People's Republic of China
e-mail: luohm@chinacdc.cn

W. Yang (ed.), *Prevention and Control of Infectious Diseases in BRI Countries*,
https://doi.org/10.1007/978-981-33-6958-0_4

annual cases reported from 2015 to 2018 (74 in 2015, 37 in 2016, 22 in 2017, 33 in 2018) [2]. Wild-type virus-caused polio outbreaks occurred in Cote d'Ivoire, Pakistan, China, Niger, Somalia, Syria, Cameroon, Equatorial Guinea, South Sudan, Madagascar, Nigeria, and Iran from 2011 to 2019. Polio vaccine-derived virus circulations were reported in Ukraine, Laos, Myanmar, Nigeria, Syria, Congo, Somalia, Papua New Guinea, Niger, Mozambique, Indonesia, Cameroon, Ghana, Philippines, China, and Pakistan from 2011 to 2019 [3].

As no WPV2 had been detected since 1999, and given the ongoing cVDPV due to the low coverage of tOPV, the connection of 26–31% of VAPP cases with the type 2 vaccine strains in the tOPV, the global immunization strategy on polio was changed in 2016, i.e., type 2 vaccine was canceled, tOPV was replaced by bOPV (including type 1 and type 2), and IPV was introduced. However, type 2 cVDPV increased beyond the estimation, indicating new challenges for polio eradication. The annual cases of type 1 cVDPV from AFP were 20, 3, 0, 27, and 6 from 2015 to 2019 (by October 15), respectively, and the annual cases of type 2 cVDPV, 12, 2, 96, 71, and 89, respectively. Central African (10), Congo (34), Nigeria (16), and Angola (18) topped the list [4]. The annual cases of type 2 cVDPV, of the same period, from the healthy population or close contacts, were 0, 3, 85, 77, and 97, respectively (by October 15, 2019).

4.1.2 Risk Assessment and Principles of Prevention and Control

4.1.2.1 Risk Assessment

The risk factors of polio infections include lack of vaccination, living in or traveling to areas with wild polio circulation, close contact with patients, and poor sanitation.

Most countries have eliminated polio through mass vaccination campaigns, but it is still prevalent in Afghanistan, Pakistan, and Nigeria, and countries like Equatorial Guinea, Guinea, Iran, Iraq, Kenya, Laos, Liberia, Madagascar, Sierra Leone, South Sudan, Syria, and Ukraine face a high risk of reemergence [5]. The potential of polio vaccine-derived virus circulation is high in many countries, which may even lead to long-distance transmission and human infection.

China achieved the goal of wild poliovirus eradication in 2000, but polio vaccine-derived viruses can circulate in people and long-distance transmission by a healthy population may occur. Before the eradication of polio worldwide, China still faces the risk of the imported wild virus in China, and once the imported virus spreads, it may also cause disease in older children or even adults [6].

4.1.2.2 Principles of Prevention and Control

To maintain a sensitive AFP surveillance system, high coverage of the polio vaccine and rapid response to the polio outbreak are the key strategies to achieve the goal of polio eradication.

4.1.2.2.1 Prevention

Children (travelers) should be vaccinated with bOPV and IPV according to the immunization program or vaccination instructions. If one wants to travel to or work in countries with polio-endemic, one dose of bOPV or IPV is recommended.

Follow tips to refrain from exposure to food or drinks that could be contaminated by the feces of a person infected with polio.

1. Eat cooked and hot food, food from sealed packages, hard-cooked eggs, fruits and vegetables washed in safe water or peeled, and dairy products pasteurized.
2. Don't eat cold dish, food served by street vendors, raw or soft-cooked eggs, raw or undercooked meat or fish, unpeeled or unwashed raw vegetables and fruits, condiments made with fresh ingredients, salads, flavored ice or popsicles, unpasteurized dairy products, and bushmeat (monkeys, bats, or other wild game).
3. Drink only bottled and sealed water, sports drinks, or sodas, water that has been disinfected (boiled, filtered), ice made with bottled or disinfected water, hot coffee or tea, and pasteurized milk.

4.1.2.2.2 Case Management

Isolate patients until resolution of illness. No specific antiviral therapy available. Supportive care is the mainstay of treatment, focusing on pain control, fever control, and physical therapy. Mechanical ventilation may be needed for respiratory failure in severe cases.

4.1.2.2.3 Outbreak Management [9]

1. Detection, notification, and investigation. Samples collected from human or environmental sources by routine surveillance or an outbreak or event are sent to a laboratory for poliovirus testing. Country informs health authorities, IHR focal point notifies WHO, and WHO headquarters inform relevant Global Polio Eradication Initiative partners. Local health authorities are required to initiate epidemiological/social investigation within 24 hours after receiving the poliovirus isolation report.

   The information outlined below should be collected:

   (a) Detailed case investigation of a person in isolation or contact of AFP case;
   (b) Investigation of the site of isolation from environmental surveillance;
   (c) Description of the community context of any detected isolation, regardless of source (population immunity, recent SIA performance, population features, movement, and migration routes);
   (d) Community search for additional AFP cases and investigating evidence of virus transmission, such as surveillance data, contact sampling, targeted healthy children stool testing, community household search, local health facility search, and other community outreach.

2. Risk assessment. Three risk elements are addressed by a risk assessment: virologic (high degree of genetic deviation from Sabin vaccine strain, number and nature of nucleotide changes, and expert interpretation by virologists), contextual (recent poliovirus detection or other sentinel events, the sensitivity of AFP surveillance system, high population density, low immunization coverage and population immunity, geographic access, conflict, inaccessible or hard-to-reach populations, and population movements), and risk of international transmission (border area with high population mobility, nomadic or refugee populations, cross border conflict, and international travel routes).
3. Surveillance following the investigation. Surveillance is enhanced to increase sensitivity and confidence that any ongoing person-to-person transmission of poliovirus will be rapidly detected.
4. Vaccination response. The timing and quality of the vaccination response are critically important.
5. Communication and social mobilization. Initiate a national advocacy and communication plan on community engagement, social mobilization, and general information dissemination strategies throughout the outbreak response period. Include pre-campaign awareness sessions targeting high-risk and hard-to-reach populations. Communicate proactively to ensure that communities and health workers are aware of the risks of the disease and the benefits of the vaccine.
6. Monitoring and evaluation of response.

4.1.3 Case Study of a Polio Outbreak in China

An Outbreak of Polio in Xinjiang in 2011

The last local patient with wild-type poliovirus was reported in China mainland, 1994. WHO Western Pacific region was declared to be a polio-free region in October 2000, indicating that China has achieved the goal of polio-free. But China is still at risk of importing polio cases due to the poliovirus circulating in Pakistan, Afghanistan, and other countries.

1. Background

Between July 3 and October 9, 2011, twenty-one confirmed cases with wild-type poliovirus infection were found in Xinjiang: 13 in Hetian, 6 in Kashi, 1 in Bazhou, and 1 in Akesu. Twenty-three probable cases of poliomyelitis were also found, with 19 in Hetan, 3 in Kashi, and 1 in Akesu. Of the 21 confirmed cases, 10 occurred in persons under 15 years and 11 in persons aged 15–53 years. Of the 10 children affected, 3 did not receive any tOPV, 2 received one or two doses, and 5 received more than two doses, indicating routine vaccination failure.

2.08% (14/673) of contacts of persons with acute flaccid paralysis (AFP) and 2.65% (13/491) of healthy persons in Hetian, Kashi, Bazhou, and Akesu were found to excrete the wild-type poliovirus. Three healthy students who resided in Beijing from Hetian were found to excrete wild-type poliovirus. Wild-type poliovirus was isolated from one sewage sample from Hetian and one sample of river water from Hetian.

On August 25, the presence of the wild-type poliovirus strains was confirmed in all four patients. The four strains diverged 20.9–21.3% from the VP1 region of the type 1 Sabin strain and were 99.2–99.6% homologous with one another by genetic sequencing. WHO confirmed that the outbreak was caused by a wild-type poliovirus imported from Pakistan, as the high degree of homologous nucleotide sequencing among the viruses isolated from Hetian and Pakistan [7].

2. Control Measures

2.1 Public health emergency response. China's central and local governments immediately launched the second-level emergency response on public health. The leadership and technical groups for the outbreak response had been designated by August 26, 2011, and worked on all aspects of management, technical supports, and communications. The local government convened an emergency response meeting for the poliomyelitis outbreak on August 30. More than 1000 healthcare workers had been trained in disease surveillance and emergency vaccination by August 31. More than five million doses of tOPV had been shipped by air force from Beijing to Xinjiang by September 2, the vaccination campaign was initiated in Xinjiang on September 8.

2.2 Risk assessment. OPV coverage rate was surveyed randomly among 2340 children under 5 years in five counties in Hetian as soon as the outbreak confirmation. The coverage rate of the third dose of tOPV administered through routine immunization was 78.8–90.9% among the children under 5 years in those counties.

2.3 Enhancement of surveillance. The local government implemented daily reports on cases of AFP as soon as outbreak confirmation. The AFP cases were reported notified by all public and private hospitals at the township level and above, and all population was monitored. A search for AFP cases since January 2010 was performed, and 410 cases were identified (122 children and 288 adults). 29.5% (121/410) of cases were detected through routine surveillance, and others (289/410) were found by retrospective searching. Of these 289 AFP cases, 15 were classified as clinically compatible with poliomyelitis, and 9 were diagnosed as confirmed cases based on laboratory testing.

2.4 Supplementary immunization. The targets for supplementary immunization were refined based on the epidemiologic nature of the outbreak. The target population was limited to children under 15 years in the first stage of supplementary immunization because all confirmed cases were in this age group at that time. When affected adults were subsequently confirmed, the target population was expanded to all people under 40 years. OPV was administered with/without vaccination history.

Public health education on the vaccination campaign was advocated repeatedly on television, on the radio, and in newspapers. Before vaccination campaigns began, SMSs were sent to mobile-phone subscribers and local political and religious leaders, community elders, and volunteers, inviting them to spread the key points and messages. The rural communities were warned about poliomyelitis and the risks of not being vaccinated. Information on the vaccination campaigns was delivered by community leaders door to door.

Campaigns among children were initiated in schools and kindergartens in August 2011. Each child's ear or finger was marked with indelible ink after vaccination, indicating that he/she had received vaccine. All fairs and markets had vaccination teams to cover every child in the area. Teams also checked on and vaccinated infants being kept at home door by door.

Five rounds of supplementary activities (SIAs) with 43.7 million doses of OPV were conducted in Xinjiang, August 2011–April 2012. Adults received OPV during four rounds of SIAs conducted in southern Xinjiang. Approximately 20 million doses of monovalent OPV type 1 (OPV1) were used during the third and fourth rounds. Trivalent OPV was used in the final round since it was used for routine immunization. 422 mild adverse events were reported after immunization without moderate or severe adverse events related to vaccination.

2.5 Interruption of transmission. The outbreak of imported wild-type poliovirus in Xinjiang was stopped 1.5 months after laboratory confirmation of the index case. The reported incidence of non-poliomyelitis-related AFP in Xinjiang in 2011 and 2012 exceeded two cases per 100,000 children under 15 years (based on population data from routine surveillance), and the timeless indicators of the AFP surveillance system met WHO requirements. The reported coverage rate was more than 98% for each round of SIA. Externally surveyed coverage was assessed in three randomly selected villages in each county and three randomly selected villages in each township. Samples were obtained from ten adults and ten children in these villages. The coverage rate of each round of SIA exceeded 95% in all counties.

2.6 Social mobilization. Substantial resources were required in outbreak investigation and response. China's central government and Xinjiang government allocated about $26 million, for the control of the outbreak. All authorities collaborated extensively in performing disease surveillance and reporting in schools and nurseries, producing and transporting vaccines, and transporting specimens and equipment. More than 500 public health experts were sent to support local health workers and government officials. And approximately 500,000 volunteers worked in the vaccination campaigns and assisted in improving the surveillance for acute flaccid paralysis.

3. What Can We Learn from This Outbreak?

Before wild-type poliovirus transmission is interrupted globally, poliomyelitis-free countries will continue to be at risk of the importation of the virus.

Control measures recommended by WHO were adopted to interrupt the transmission of wild-type poliovirus. Key response measures included the declaration of a public health emergency, improvement of the sensitivity of AFP surveillance, the initiation of epidemiologically targeted vaccination campaigns, the use of OPV for two rounds of SIAs, close collaboration with international agencies such as the WHO and the US CDC, and the provision of adequate resources to upgrade the responses.

Substantial efforts were required to maintain poliomyelitis-free status: high coverage rate of polio vaccines, frequent risk assessments, sensitive laboratory-supported AFP, and preparedness for outbreak detection and response. All countries will be benefited from the global eradication of poliomyelitis, including those countries that have been certified as poliomyelitis-free [7, 8].

4.2 Measles

Measles is an acute, highly contagious, and highly seasonal respiratory infectious disease caused by the measles virus. The only natural host is humans who can sustain measles virus transmission. Person-to-person transmission occurs primarily by the airborne route. The measles' symptoms appear 7–14 days after exposure and typically include a prodromal fever that can reach as high as 40 °C, conjunctivitis, coryza, cough, and small spots with white or bluish-white centers on an erythematous base on the buccal mucosa (Koplik spots). A characteristic red, blotchy (maculopapular) rash presents on the 3rd to 7th day after the occurrence of prodromal symptoms. Encephalitis occurs in approximately 1 per 1000–2000 cases, which can result in permanent brain damage. The risk of serious complications and death is the highest for children under 5 years and adults aged 20 years or above. It is quite high in populations with poor nutritional status.

4.2.1 Overview of Measles in the "Belt and Road" Countries

While global measles deaths have decreased by 84% which was from 550,100 deaths in 2000 to 89,780 deaths in 2016, measles is still common in many developing countries, particularly in parts of Africa and Asia. About seven million people were affected by measles in 2016. More than 95% of measles deaths occur in countries with low per capita incomes and weak health infrastructures [10].

According to the joint report of WHO and UNICEF, no measles cases were reported in 31 countries from 2011 to 2018. The 30 countries that top the list of reported measles from 2011 to 2018 are Congo (453,000), China (173,000), India (151,000), Nigeria (133,000), Indonesia (95,000), Philippines (94,000), Somalia (80,000), Ukraine (72,000), Pakistan (68,000), Ethiopia (52,000), Mongolia (51,000), Romania (31,000), Sudan (29,000), Angola (26,000), Madagascar (21,000), Vietnam (20,000), Thailand (20,000), Kyrgyzstan (19,000), Niger (18,000), Uganda (18,000), Yemen (18,000), France (16,000), Bangladesh (16,000), Zambia (14,000), Russia (14,000), Georgia (14,000), Burkina Faso (13,000), Italy (13,000), Chad (12,000), and Nepal (12,000). The 30 countries that top the list of annual incidence rate (per 100,000 people) are Mongolia (213.18), Congo (75.30), Somalia (73.63), Equatorial Guinea (48.78), Georgia (43.04), Kyrgyzstan (40.92), Ukraine (20.09), Liberia (19.65), Romania (19.28), Gabon (18.14), Bosnia and Herzegovina (17.72), Micronesia (16.19), Nauru (13.28), Sierra Leone (12.87), Djibouti (12.03), Angola (12.01), Philippines (11.66), Niger (11.48), Zambia (11.35), Madagascar (11.20), Chad (11.04), Namibia (10.59), Burkina Faso (9.36), Sudan (9.33), Republic of Serbia (9.28), Nigeria Leah (9.27), East Timor (9.21), Congo (Brazzaville) (8.82), Central Africa (8.79), and Yemen (8.48) [5].

The goals of eliminating measles by 2020 were established in all WHO member countries. 82 out of 194 member countries have been confirmed to have eliminated measles by 2019. Seven countries, namely Venezuela, Brazil, Mongolia, Albania, Czech Republic, and Greece, have seen local transmission of measles virus reoccurred after declaring the goal of eliminating measles, possibly for lack of political will, conflict, immigration, humanitarian emergency, insufficient national financial investment, and vaccine hesitation, making it difficult to maintain a high level of measles vaccine coverage among the population (92–94%). The high contagiousness of the measles virus constitutes one reason for the unstable elimination of measles. With the deepening of globalization and the increasingly close relationship between countries, the risk of cross-border transmission of measles persists.

In 2019, measles outbreaks reoccurred in many countries, and by November 2019, it was continuously found in Madagascar and Nigeria. 250,270 suspected cases and 5110 associated deaths in total were reported by the Democratic Republic of the Congo. 25,596 suspected cases were reported in 94% of Chad's districts. Current outbreaks of concern include Yemen with 5847 confirmed cases, Sudan (3659), Somalia (2795), Pakistan (1978), Tunisia (1367), and Iraq (1222). Ukraine has reported 56,802 cases, followed by Kazakhstan (10,126), Georgia (3904), Russia (3521), Turkey (2666), and Kyrgyzstan (2228). Brazil has reported 11,887 confirmed cases, with the majority of cases in Sao Paulo. Bangladesh has reported 4181 confirmed cases of measles. Myanmar, Thailand, and Bangladesh in Southeast Asia have reported 5286, 4852, and 4181 confirmed cases, respectively. New Zealand has reported 2084 confirmed cases, of which 80% are in the Auckland region. There were outbreaks of measles in Tonga, Fiji, and American Samoa [11].

4.2.2 Risk Assessment and Principles of Prevention and Control

4.2.2.1 Risk Assessment

Measles is a highly contagious viral disease which affects susceptible individuals of all ages and remains one of the leading causes of death among young children globally, despite the availability of safe and effective measles-containing vaccines.

Despite the implementation of routine immunization, measles continues to circulate globally due to suboptimal vaccination coverage and population immunity gaps. Community having immunity level less than 95% would face the risk of an outbreak. The coverage of the first dose of measles vaccine is below 80% in Equatorial Guinea, Samoa, Papua New Guinea, South Sudan, Gabon, Lesotho, Nigeria, Pakistan, Philippines, Bosnia and Herzegovina-Serbia, Chad, Somalia, Cameroon, Central Africa, Mali, Yemen, Micronesia, Benin, Haiti, Venezuela, Guinea, Vanuatu, Niger, East Timor, Angola, Guinea-Bissau, Kenya, and Laos in 2018. Without a timely and comprehensive response to an outbreak, the virus will contact vulnerable individuals and potentially spread within and beyond the affected areas.

The impact on public health will persist unless the ongoing outbreaks are controlled, routine vaccination coverage remains more than 95%, and immunity gaps in the population are filled. As long as measles continues to circulate in the world, no country can be assured to be free of importation. However, countries can protect their populations through high vaccine coverage primarily by routine immunization programs and supplemental immunization activities designed to assure that susceptible individuals are vaccinated [11].

4.2.2.2 Principles of Prevention and Control

The basic strategy to control and eliminate measles is to achieve and maintain high-level coverage of measles vaccine of two doses.

4.2.2.2.1 Prevention

Children (travelers) should be vaccinated with measles vaccines. One dose of measles vaccine is recommended to travelers and workers, which have not been infected or vaccinated, in countries with the measles epidemic.

Maintain hygiene and sanitation. Wash your hands often with soap and water. If those aren't available, clean your hands with hand sanitizer (at least 60% alcohol). Avoid touching your eyes, nose, or mouth. If need to touch your face, clean your hands. Cover your mouth and nose with a tissue or your sleeve when coughing or sneezing. Maintain good indoor ventilation [12].

4.2.2.2.2 Case Management

Infected people should be isolated for 4 days after rash onset. Airborne precautions should be followed in healthcare settings. There is no specific antiviral therapy for measles. Severe complications from measles can be reduced through supportive care, such as good nutrition, adequate fluid intake, and treatment of dehydration with oral rehydration solution. This solution replaces fluids and other essential elements that can be lost through diarrhea or vomiting. Eye and ear infections, and pneumonia can be treated by antibiotics.

4.2.2.2.3 Outbreak Management

1. Manage cases and contacts to control spread. Health staff should report all suspect patients with measles. Limit contact only to immediate family members who have been vaccinated or have a history of measles confirmed by healthcare workers. Avoid contact with infants or young unimmunized children in the household. Patients with measles who require hospitalization should be isolated from the onset of prodromal symptoms until 5 days after rash onset. Health staff in contact with patients should follow respiratory precautions. Close contacts without documented evidence of measles vaccination should be immunized and the symptoms of measles should be informed. During the 2nd week after exposure, and at the first possible sign of measles (fever, runny nose, cough, or red eyes), the contacts should be required to stay at home.
2. Conduct appropriate vaccination activities. Once the decision to intervene is made, act as quickly as possible to reduce the number of severe measles cases and deaths. First, enhance social mobilization to inform the suspected outbreak-affected communities, the target age group of previously unvaccinated children, and the points of vaccine that parents should bring their at-risk children for vaccination. Second, vaccinate all target children based on the local disease epidemiology without a history of measles vaccination in health facilities or at outreach vaccination sites. Third, vaccinate hospital staff who have not been vaccinated and thus at risk of exposure. Fourth, guarantee sufficient supplies. Use stock management records to determine the available quantity and location of vaccines, auto-disable syringes, cold-chain equipment, and other supplies that are immediately available. Estimate and request the additional supplies needed timely so that activities would not be interrupted due to supply stock-out.
3. Ensure effective community involvement and public awareness. When an outbreak is confirmed, it is likely to arouse widespread public concern and attract media attention. Keep the public well informed, ask them to stay calm, and encourage cooperation. Clear and concise messages should be delivered to the community [13].

4.3 Meningococcal Disease

Meningococcal disease refers to any illness caused by bacteria called *Neisseria meningitidis*, also known as meningococcus. These illnesses are often severe or deadly. They include infections of the lining of the brain and spinal cord (meningitis) and bloodstream infections (bacteremia or septicemia).

The most common symptoms of meningococcal meningitis include fever, headache, and stiff neck. Nausea, vomiting, photophobia, and confusion are also commonly seen. Newborns and babies may be slow or inactive, irritable, vomit, feed poorly, or have a bulging in the soft spot of the skull. Symptoms of meningococcal septicemia may include fever and chills, fatigue, vomiting, cold hands and feet, severe aches or pain in the muscles, joints, chest, or abdomen, rapid breathing, diarrhea, etc.

Neisseria meningitidis only infects humans; there is no animal reservoir. Human is generally susceptive to the bacteria. *Neisseria meningitidis* is transmitted from person to person through droplets of respiratory or throat secretions from carriers. Close and prolonged contact facilitates the spread of the disease, such as kissing, sneezing, coughing on someone, or living in close quarters (such as a dormitory, sharing eating, or drinking utensils) with an infected person.

Neisseria meningitidis is classified into 12 serogroups (A, B, C, 29E, H, I, K, L, W135, X, Y, and Z) based on the structure of the polysaccharide capsule.

4.3.1 Overview of Meningococcal Diseases in the "Belt and Road" Countries

Meningococcal disease is found worldwide. Global pandemics have been caused by group A *Neisseria meningitis*. The Global Burden of Disease estimated the incidence of Meningococcal diseases at 23.3 per 100,000 in 2015 [15]. The highest incidence occurs in the "Meningitis Belt" of sub-Saharan Africa, stretching from Senegal in the west to Ethiopia in the east.

The meningococcal diseases were reported in Congo (6012), Nigeria (4516), Burkina Faso (2421), Niger (1496), Cameroon (1060), Ghana (987), Mali (755), Togo (683), Central Africa (467), Chad (401), Guinea (353), Benin (322), Uganda (231), Kenya (196), Senegal (195), South Sudan (37), Tanzania (22), and Gambia (19), in the "Meningitis Belt" in 2018 [16].

According to statistics of WHO, based on the serogroup distribution of invasive meningococcal diseases, in 2018, the predominant *Neisseria meningitis* are serogroup B, C, and W in Asia and Europe, serogroup A and C in the Mediterranean, serogroup B and C in Australia and South America, serogroup B, C, and Y in North America, serogroup B in North Africa, serogroup C, W, and X in the "Meningitis Belt" and serogroup B and W in South Africa [6].

4.3.2 Risk Assessment and Principles of Prevention and Control

4.3.2.1 Risk Assessment

The cluster and small-scale outbreaks of meningococcal diseases still occur with seasonal changes globally. Meningococcal diseases occur mainly in the "Meningitis Belt". Since 2010 and the roll-out of a meningococcal A conjugate vaccine through mass preventive immunization campaigns in the "Meningitis Belt", the proportion of A serogroup has declined dramatically, and outbreaks caused by serogroup of W, X, and C are low in frequency and scale [17].

4.3.2.2 Principles of Prevention and Control

4.3.2.2.1 Prevention

Group A, Group AC, and Group ACYW meningococcal vaccines are approved in China. Group B meningococcal vaccine is available in the world. Children (travelers) should be vaccinated according to the schedule of immunization programs or vaccine instructions.

Maintain standards of hygiene and sanitation. Wash your hands often with soap and water. If those aren't available, clean hands with hand sanitizer (containing at least 60% alcohol). Don't touch your eyes, nose, or mouth. Cover your mouth and nose with a tissue or your sleeve when coughing or sneezing. Maintain good indoor ventilation.

Do regular and appropriate physical exercises and outdoor activities. Eat a balanced diet. Keep enough rest and sleep. Keep children away from patients with meningococcal diseases. Wear masks in crowded places in epidemic season. If fever, headache, and vomiting occur, visit the doctor as soon as possible. Vaccinate with meningococcal vaccines.

4.3.2.2.2 Case Management

A number of antibiotics are chosen by doctors to treat meningococcal disease. It is important that treatment starts as soon as possible. On suspecting the meningococcal disease, the doctor should give the patient antibiotics immediately. Antibiotics can decrease the risk of dying. Depending on how serious the infection is, people with meningococcal disease may need other treatments, including breathing support, medications to treat low blood pressure, surgery to remove dead tissue, and wound care for parts of the body with damaged skin.

4.3.2.2.3 Close Contacts Management

People in the same household, roommates, and anyone with direct contact with the patient's saliva should be considered as close contacts. Close contacts should receive antimicrobial chemoprophylaxis as early as possible. Close contacts should receive medical observation for more than 7 days from the last contact and be told to minimize contact with others. If sudden shiver, high fever, nausea, vomiting, runny nose, sore throat, general pain, headache, or ecchymosis occur, they should visit doctors as soon as possible.

Before potential protection from vaccination, chemoprophylaxis can be used as an interim measure to temporarily reduce meningococcal carriage and transmission. When making decisions to implement chemoprophylaxis, consider the appropriate target group, the feasibility of antibiotic administration to all target persons within the shortest time (ideally within 24 h), and risk of exposure due to multiple sources of transmission within a population during the outbreak [18].

4.3.2.2.4 Outbreak Control

Enhance meningococcal surveillance during the outbreak. Healthcare providers and laboratories should be informed to be vigilant of patients with symptoms suggestive of meningococcal disease if a suspected outbreak occurs. They should ensure that all suspected cases of meningococcal disease to be reported to the local health department and that any subsequent suspected cases are promptly reported.

Vaccinate people identified with increased risk. The vaccine depends on the serogroup causing the outbreak. In outbreaks caused by serogroup A, C, W, or Y, inject people of 2 months and above and identified with increased risk of Group AC or Group ACYW meningococcal conjugate vaccines.

Keep communities and healthcare personnel adequately informed of meningococcal disease, and promote early care-seeking behaviors and disease recognition, which are important for managing suspected meningococcal disease outbreaks. Health education should be initiated as soon as a suspected outbreak of meningococcal disease is reported.

Restrict travel to an area with an outbreak, close schools or universities, or cancel sporting or social events.

The rooms where patients live and work should be disinfected with chlorinated disinfectants.

4.3.3 Control of Meningococcal Diseases in the "Meningitis Belt"

Control of Meningococcal Diseases in the "Meningitis Belt"

1. Background

Meningococcal diseases have been prevalent in Africa for more than 100 years. It is possible that the meningococcal diseases were introduced by pilgrims from Sudan to West Africa. Meningococcal outbreaks occurred every a few years in sub-Saharan Africa. About 200,000 cases were reported in 1996 [19]. The largest burden of meningococcal disease occurred in an area of sub-Saharan Africa (known as the Meningitis Belt), which stretches from Senegal in the west to Ethiopia in the east and covers 26 countries.

During the dry season between December and June, dust winds, cold nights, and upper respiratory tract infections combine to damage the nasopharyngeal mucosa which were the risk factors for meningococcal disease. At the same time, the transmission of *Neisseria meningitis* may be facilitated by overcrowded housing [14].

2. Control Measures

2.1 Establish the roadmap to defeat meningitis by 2030. A global strategy to "defeat meningitis by 2030" is being prepared by a WHO-led multi-organization technical taskforce. The vision of the roadmap is a world free of meningitis. The goals proposed to be achieved by 2030 are: (1) eliminate meningitis epidemics; (2) reduce the number of cases and deaths from vaccine-preventable meningitis by 80%; (3) decrease the impact of sequelae by 50%. The strategy will be based on five pillars: prevention and epidemic control, diagnosis and treatment, disease surveillance, support and care for patients and their families, and advocacy and engagement.

2.2 Launch the pediatric bacterial meningitis (PBM) surveillance network. PBM network is launched by WHO and global immunization partners in the WHO-African Region in 2001 to collect information on laboratory-confirmed bacterial meningitis cases among children under 5 years at sentinel hospitals. The number of countries involved in the network increased from 8 in 2003 to 24 in 2018.

2.3 Conduct mass vaccination campaigns. The International Coordinating Group (ICG) on Vaccine Provision for Epidemic Meningitis Control was established in January 1997, following major outbreaks of meningitis in Africa. ICG is made up of four member agencies: IFRC, MSF, UNICEF, and WHO. From 2009 to 2016, twenty million doses of vaccines were shipped for emergency response in thirteen countries. Before 2010, serogroup A was responsible for most epidemics. Starting in 2010, a meningococcal A conjugate vaccine was introduced progressively into epidemic-prone areas in countries of African's Meningitis Belt through mass preventive vaccination campaigns. This has dramatically reduced the number of *Neisseria meningitis*. In total, 8 of the 26 Meningitis Belt countries have now introduced the vaccine into their routine immunization program.

2.4 Make standard operating procedures (SOPs) for surveillance of meningitis and preparedness and response to epidemics in Africa. The third updated version of the SOPs was issued by WHO in October 2018. It includes recommended practices for both enhanced and case-based surveillance. The aim of the SOPs for meningitis surveillance, preparedness, and response to epidemics in Africa is to guide health personnel at various levels of the health system in the implementation of enhanced and, where relevant, case-based surveillance of meningitis and in prompt response to meningitis epidemics.

2.5 Response to outbreaks. The main measure to respond to the meningitis outbreak is mass vaccination, with funding and vaccine support from international organizations.

3. What We Can Learn from the Meningitis Belt?

WHO has worked with relevant countries to conduct mass vaccination campaigns with Group A meningococcal vaccines and introduced them into the national immunization program. The number of serogroup A meningitis cases has dropped to the lowest level in Africa. But if related countries stop the vaccination with Group A meningococcal vaccines, the outbreak will reoccur.

There is an increasing trend of serotype W, X, and C meningitis diseases and outbreaks in the Meningitis Belt. Therefore, it is necessary to introduce serotype ACYW meningococcal vaccines to the Meningitis Belt.

4.4 Japanese Encephalitis

Japanese encephalitis (JE) virus is the leading cause of vaccine-preventable encephalitis in Asia and the Western Pacific. JE virus exists in a transmission cycle between mosquitoes, pigs, and/or water birds. Humans who are bitten by an infected mosquito can be infected, such as *Culex* mosquito, *Aedes* mosquito, and *Anopheles* mosquito. JE predominantly occurs in rural and periurban settings. Most JE virus infections are mild (fever and headache) or inapparent, but approximately 0.5% of infections results in severe disease with rapid onset of high fever, headache, neck stiffness, disorientation, coma, seizures, spastic paralysis, and death. The case-fatality rate can be more than 30% among those with disease symptoms, and 20–30% of survivors suffer permanent neuropsychiatric sequelae. In areas where the JE virus is common, encephalitis occurs mainly in young children due to older children and adults already infected and with immune [20].

4.4.1 Overview of JE in the "Belt and Road" Countries

According to the joint report of WHO and UNICEF, from 2011 to 2018, JE cases were not reported in 171 countries, but cumulative cases of JE were reported in China (11,125), followed in number by India (10,946), Nepal (2778), Vietnam (2192), Bangladesh (1846), Myanmar (1161), Philippines (1085), Indonesia (436), Thailand (287), Cambodia (275), Sri Lanka (268), Malaysia (236), Laos (112), South Korea (112), Bhutan (46), Japan (38), East Timor (13), Australia (10), Papua New Guinea (6), Sweden (3), Brunei (2), Norway (1), and Czech Republic (1). The annual incidence (per 10,000 people) of JE was reported in Nepal (1.28), followed by Bhutan (0.80), Vietnam (0.30), Myanmar (0.28), Cambodia (0.22), Laos (0.21), Sri Lanka (0.16), Bangladesh (0.15), East Timor (0.14), Philippines (0.13), India (0.11), China (0.10), Malaysia (0.10), Brunei (0.06), Thailand (0.05), South Korea (0.03), Indonesia (0.02), Papua New Guinea (0.009), Australia (0.005), Sweden (0.004), Japan (0.004), Norway (0.002), and Czech Republic (0.001) [5].

4.4.2 Risk Assessment and Principles of Prevention and Control

4.4.2.1 Risk Assessment

JE commonly occurs throughout most of Asia and parts of the Western Pacific. Transmission occurs principally in rural agricultural areas and is often associated with rice cultivation and flood irrigation. These ecologic conditions may appear near or within urban centers in some areas of Asia. The transmission is seasonal in temperate areas of Asia, and the human disease usually peaks in summer and fall. Seasonal transmission varies with monsoon rains and irrigation practices, and may be prolonged or even occur year-round in the subtropics and tropics.

In endemic countries where adults have already acquired immunity through natural infection, JE occurs mainly in children. Travelers that go to Asia are at risk of getting JE. For most travelers, the risk is extremely low (less than one case per one million) but it varies with the destination, duration, season, and activities. Expatriates and travelers are at higher risk if they stay at places of the epidemic, travel a long time there, or are involved in a number of outdoor activities in rural areas in a time of active transmission [21].

4.4.2.2 Principles of Prevention and Control

4.4.2.2.1 Prevention

Children (travelers) should be vaccinated with the JE live-attenuated or inactivated vaccine.

Avoid mosquito bites. Cover exposed skin by wearing long-sleeved shirts, long pants, and hats. Use an appropriate insect repellent as directed. Longer protection can be provided by higher percentages of active ingredients. Use permethrin-treated clothing and gear (such as boots, pants, socks, and tents). Stay and sleep in screened or air-conditioned rooms. Use a bed net if the area where you are sleeping is exposed to the outdoors.

4.4.2.2.2 Cases Management

There are no specific treatments found for patients with JE, but hospitalization for supportive care and close observation is generally required.

Treatment is symptomatic. Rest, fluids, and use of pain relievers and medication to reduce fever may relieve some symptoms.

4.4.2.2.3 Outbreak Control [22]

Patients should be diagnosed and treated early. JE-confirmed and -suspected cases should be investigated by public health workers. Blood or cerebrospinal fluid samples should be collected for laboratory testing.

Conduct an active case search to definitude the actual epidemic size. Analyze the epidemic factors.

Conduct health education on the prevention and control of JE.

Reduce mosquitos, especially for children, with public health insecticide.

Conduct emergency vaccination. Identify the immunization areas, target population, and implementation time, according to the epidemic characteristics and immunity of residents.

4.4.3 Prevention and Control of JE in China

Japanese Encephalitis Control in China

1. Background

JE-suspected cases have been found since 1922. JE virus was identified in a serological test in 1934. It was isolated from the brain tissue of a dead person in Beijing in 1940. The incidence of JE increased year by year in the 1950s, similar to the trends in Japan and South Korea. The first peak of JE appeared in 1957, with 34,245 cases, 8075 deaths, and a case fatality rate of 23.58%. The infection status of JE among the health population was surveyed in more than 30 cities. The recessive infection rates were high, such as in Shenyang (71%) and Jinzhou (52%) in the north, indicating that the JE virus was widespread in China. For other peaks of JE, one appeared in 1966 (151,251 cases and the incidence of 20.58 per 100,000) and one in 1971 (174,932 cases and the incidence of 20.92 per 100,000). The endemic area expended, including north and east of inner Mongolia, and Northwest China [23]. Thanks to the wide use of JE vaccines and the control of mosquitos, the incidence of JE saw a yearly decrease, dropping to <10 per 100,000 in the mid-1970s and <5 per 100,000 in the 1980s. Currently, it is about <0.5 per 100,000.

2. Control Measures

The main prevention strategy was to provide JE vaccination to children and adults. Surveillance of JE cases, vectors, hosts, and outbreak management was also enhanced.

Develop the JE vaccine, incorporate it into the national immunization program, and carry out mass vaccination for the risk population in the endemic areas. Professor Yu Yongxin invented firstly the live attenuated vaccine through the SA 14-14-2 strain, with highly weakened virulence, good immunogenicity, and high genetic stability. The vaccine was approved in 1989 and widely used in the whole country. JE vaccines were included in China's immunization program in 2008. Children were routinely vaccinated with JE vaccines in China, except Tibet, Qinghai, and Xinjiang. To prevent the possible outbreak of JE after the Wenchuan 8.0 Richter scale earthquake, children were vaccinated in shelters and schools of the earthquake-stricken area in Sichuan, Gansu, and Shaanxi. The coverage of JE vaccines was 95.29% in Sichuan, 95.95% in Gansu, 98.48% in Shaanxi, as was shown in quick field investigations. The massive vaccination of JE vaccines was conducted in 308 counties of 12 provinces in 2018, where the incidence of JE was more than 1 per 100,000. The overall coverage was above 90%. The incidence of the target population in the 308 counties got lower after massive vaccination. The number of JE cases decreased by 73.62%.

Enhance the surveillance and laboratory test of JE cases and conduct surveillance of mosquitos, vectors, and hosts. The report of JE cases and prevention measures was specified in 1955. The internet- and case-based surveillance have been conducted since 2004. The national workshop and laboratory test training was conducted annually. The sentinel surveillance was initiated in 2005 for case surveillance, improving laboratory test rate, and the surveillance of mosquitos, serological surveillance of hosts, and healthy population. China CDC became a member of the WHO Western Pacific JE Reference Laboratory and set up provincial JE Reference Laboratory Network in China.

Tackle the JE outbreak in time. Local governments where the JE outbreak occurred organized CDCs, hospitals, and communities to rapidly carry out field investigations and medical treatments. Public health campaigns on mosquito control were conducted. Health education was offered through mass media on JE prevention and control. Unvaccinated people were encouraged to receive the JE vaccine.

The development of the social economy and the improvement of health conditions help reduce the incidence of JE. In recent years, the living standards of people have significantly improved; humans and livestock are separated; pigs and other livestock have gradually shifted from free-range to large-scale farming; there is extensive use of insecticides, mosquito repellents, and mosquito nets. The above-mentioned changes have reduced the risk of JE in residences.

3. What Can We Learn from China?

JE vaccine is the most effective prevention and control measure. The experience of prevention and control of JE in China shows that the most effective immunization strategy in JE endemic area is a one-time campaign in the primary target population defined by local epidemiology, followed by adding JE vaccine into the routine childhood immunization program.

JE is a zoonotic disease that cannot be eliminated in the natural environment. It is still a major threat to the health of people, and the prevention and control of it should always be paid attention to.

4.5 Diphtheria

Diphtheria is an acute respiratory infection caused by the bacterium *Corynebacterium diphtheriae,* which is a great dead threat to the human in history and primarily infects the throat and upper airways and produces a toxin affecting other organs. Humans are a reservoir for transmission. Most of the adult carriers are asymptomatic. Person-to-person transmission through respiratory droplets, close physical contact, and by fomites. Cutaneous diphtheria can be transmitted by contact with skin lesions rarely. Respiratory diphtheria includes pharyngeal and tonsillar diphtheria (most common form; typically presents with sore throat, anorexia, malaise, and low-grade fever; noticeable bluish-white membrane on palate, tonsil, or at the back of throat; neck may be swollen due to marked edema of neighboring tissue and lymphadenopathy; profound systemic illness may develop due to absorption of large amounts of the toxin), anterior nasal diphtheria (typically presents with symptoms like the common cold; a nasal discharge may be mucous or purulent or bleed; whitish membrane may be seen on nasal septum; systemic illness is uncommon as a minimal toxin), and laryngeal diphtheria (typically present with fever, hoarseness, and cough; airway obstruction may result from membrane formation and inflammatory response).

4.5.1 Overview of Diphtheria in the "Belt and Road" Countries

Diphtheria occurs around the world with a higher prevalence in temperate climates area and rare in developed countries with high qualified routine vaccination. Diphtheria mainly threatens the pre-school and school-age children in the endemic areas. With the diphtheria-containing vaccines used widely, the incidence of diphtheria decreased rapidly. There have been no diphtheria cases reported in Europe and the USA for more than 10 years, and the cases have also decreased in the developing countries yearly. An outbreak of diphtheria was reported in Russia and the former Soviet republics, with 125,000 cases (90% of the global cases) and 4000 deaths. The causes of the outbreak included the socioeconomic instability, deterioration of basic sanitation facilities, no diphtheria-containing vaccines and antitoxins supplied from Russia for the newly independent countries, improper handling contraindications, vaccination hesitancy, etc., the coverage rate of the diphtheria-containing vaccine was low, and the susceptibility increased with the reducing the immunity induced by adults vaccines.

Endemic occurred in many countries in Asia, Middle East, South Pacific, and Eastern Europe. Respiratory diphtheria outbreaks have occurred in Indonesia, Bangladesh, Myanmar, Vietnam, Venezuela, Haiti, South Africa, and Yemen. Cutaneous diphtheria has occurred commonly in tropical countries. Diphtheria can affect any population with different ages [24].

According to the WHO and UNICEF joint report, there was no diphtheria case reported in 121 countries from 2011 to 2018. The top 20 countries with cumulative cases of diphtheria were India (35,811), Indonesia (5525), Madagascar (4498), Yemen (2648), Nepal (2540), Nigeria (1870), Venezuela (1592), Pakistan (1306), Iran (673), Myanmar (511), Laos (357), Philippines (308), Thailand (268), Sudan (224), Haiti (223), Central Africa (189), Niger (122), Viet Nam (114), Bangladesh (91), and Malaysia (91). The top 20 countries with an average annual incidence (per 100,000 population) of diphtheria were Madagascar (2.35), Yemen (1.27), Nepal (1.17), Venezuela (0.67), Laos (0.67), Central Africa (0.52), Latvia (0.39), India (0.34), Indonesia (0.27), Haiti (0.26), Nigeria (0.13), Myanmar (0.12), Iran (0.11), Pakistan (0.08), Eritrea (0.08), Niger (0.08), Sudan (0.07), Somalia (0.07), New Zealand (0.07), and Samoa (0.06) [5].

4.5.2 Risk Assessment and Principles of Prevention and Control

4.5.2.1 Risk Assessment

The morbidity and mortality of diphtheria have significantly reduced since the wide vaccination on diphtheria-containing vaccines. Diphtheria is still a threat to children in countries with a low coverage rate of diphtheria-containing vaccines. The scatter or outbreak of diphtheria often occurs in endemic areas. The case-fatality rate is about 5–10%, and the rate among children is higher than among other populations.

The risk of diphtheria scatter and outbreak is high among countries with political instability or low economic development levels, such as Samoa, Equatorial Guinea, South Sudan, Papua New Guinea, Nigeria, Venezuela, Philippines, Syria, Somalia, Ukraine, Gabon, Mali, Pakistan, Bosnia and Herzegovina, Central Africa, Guinea, Micronesia, Vietnam, Indonesia, Paraguay, Chad, Cameroon, Haiti, Niger, and Uganda. The coverage rates of the third dose of diphtheria-containing vaccines were less than 80% among the above-mentioned countries in 2018.

4.5.2.2 Principles of Prevention and Control

4.5.2.2.1 Prevention

Children (travelers) should be vaccinated with diphtheria-containing vaccines, according to the schedule of immunization program and vaccine specifications in the countries of residence.

Maintain standards of hygiene and sanitation. Wash your hands often with soap and water. If those aren't available, clean your hands with hand sanitizer (at least 60% alcohol). Avoiding touching your eyes, nose, or mouth. Cover your mouth and nose with a tissue or your sleeve when coughing or sneezing. Maintain good indoor ventilation.

4.5.2.2.2 Cases Management

Patients diagnosed as diphtheria require hospitalization in respiratory isolation to monitor response to treatment and manage complications.

Patients should be treated with antitoxin and antibiotics. Equine diphtheria antitoxin is the mainstay of treatment and can be administered without laboratory confirmation. A sensitive antibiotic should be used to eliminate the causative organisms, interrupt exotoxin production, and reduce communicability, such as erythromycin or penicillin.

Aggressive supportive care may be needed, including close monitoring for respiratory compromise, mechanical ventilation.

The terminal disinfection should be conducted in the patient's houses and wards after their releasing from isolation and discharging from hospitals.

4.5.2.2.3 Close Contacts Management

Close contacts include family members and other persons with a history of direct contact with diphtheria patients, and healthcare workers who are exposed to the patients' oral or respiratory secretions.

Close contacts should receive 7-day medical observation. They can be released from medical observation after their asymptomatic characters and negative result of nasopharyngeal culture. Carriers should be placed in respiratory isolation and provided antibiotics.

Adult close contacts should avoid contacting their children and are not allowed to work in the food preparation unless releasing observation.

Close contacts should be provided with post-exposure prophylaxis. They should receive an age-appropriate diphtheria-containing vaccine, especially among the risk population (healthcare workers and caregivers) and adults aged under 45 years without diphtheria-containing vaccination within 3 years. Antimicrobial prophylaxis is recommended for close contacts, such as erythromycin or penicillin.

4.6 Hepatitis A

Hepatitis A is a vaccine-preventable and communicable disease of the liver caused by the hepatitis A virus. Symptoms usually occur abruptly and include fever, fatigue, loss of appetite, nausea, vomiting, abdominal pain, dark urine, diarrhea, clay-colored stool, joint pain, and jaundice (yellowing in sclera, skin, and urine). Most of the patients do not have symptoms or have unrecognized infections. Hepatitis A is transmitted primarily by the fecal–oral route, that is, by ingesting contaminated food and water, or through direct contact with an infectious person. The main source of infection are patients with hepatitis A and recessive infection. Human beings are susceptible to the hepatitis A virus. Almost everyone recovers fully from hepatitis A with lifelong immunity. The risk of hepatitis A outbreak is associated with poor sanitation, hygiene, and low economic level.

4.6.1 Overview of Hepatitis A in the "Belt and Road" Countries

Globally, there are an estimated 1.4 million cases of hepatitis A every year [25].

Areas with a high level of infection are India, Pakistan, Bangladesh in South Asia, the Democratic Republic of the Congo, Angola, Ethiopia, Tanzania, Sudan, South Africa, Zimbabwe, Namibia, Nigeria, Ghana, and Côte d'Ivoire in Africa. The above-mentioned low- and middle-income countries have poor sanitary conditions and hygienic habits, and the infection in these countries is common. Most children (90%) are infected with the hepatitis A virus before 10 years, and most of these infected show no symptoms. Epidemics of hepatitis A are uncommon among older children and adults as most of them have developed immunity against hepatitis A. Symptomatic disease rates in these areas are low and outbreaks are rare.

Areas with low levels of infection: Western Pacific Area (Japan, South Korea, Singapore, Australia, New Zealand, China, Indonesia, Philippines, Vietnam), America (USA, Canada, Cuba, Dominican Republic, Haiti), Europe (Germany, France, UK, Poland, Romania, Russia, Ukraine, Belarus). The above-mentioned high-income countries have good sanitary and hygienic conditions. Hepatitis A may occur among adolescents and adults in high-risk groups, such as injection drug users, MSM, people traveling to high endemic areas, and isolated populations (like closed religious groups). A large outbreak among homeless persons was reported in the USA. 3813 cases of hepatitis A among MSM were reported in 22 European countries from June 1, 2016 to December 18, 2017 [26].

Areas with intermediate levels of infection are Europe (Uzbekistan, Kazakhstan, Azerbaijan), America (Peru, Ecuador, Bolivia, Mexico, Colombia, Venezuela, Argentina, Chile, Uruguay, Brazil, Paraguay), Mediterranean (Egypt, Iran, Turkey), and Western Pacific Area (Papua New Guinea, Fiji, Solomon Islands). The above-mentioned middle-income countries and areas have unstable health status and sanitary conditions. Children are often uninfected at an early stage and have no corresponding immunity when they grow up. This higher susceptibility among older age groups may lead to a higher incidence of hepatitis and large outbreaks can occur in these communities [25, 27].

4.6.2 Risk Assessment and Principles of Prevention and Control

4.6.2.1 Risk Assessment

Hepatitis A infection is usually acute and self-limiting, and in general, does not cause chronic liver diseases. A small number of patients develop severe symptoms that last for several months. Anyone who has not been vaccinated or previously infected can get infected with the hepatitis A virus. In areas where the virus is widespread (high endemicity), most hepatitis A infections occur when people are in their early childhood. People at increased risk of hepatitis A include those traveling to or working in countries with intermediate-to-high endemicity of infection, those in child care centers and schools, MSM, persons who are homeless, users of injection and noninjecting illicit drugs, persons who work with hepatitis A virus-infected primates or with hepatitis A virus in research laboratories, persons who are administered clotting-factor concentrates, persons with chronic liver diseases (including those with chronic hepatitis B virus and chronic hepatitis C virus infection), food-service establishments or food handlers, persons currently or recently incarcerated, and workers exposed to sewage [24, 28].

4.6.2.2 Principles of Prevention and Control

4.6.2.2.1 Prevention

Children (travelers) should be vaccinated according to the schedule of immunization programs and instructions of the hepatitis A vaccine.

Maintain good hygiene and sanitation. Wash your hands often with soap and water. If those aren't available, clean your hands with hand sanitizer (at least 60% alcohol). Avoid close contact, such as kissing, hugging, or sharing eating utensils or cups with people who are sick.

Food safety. Eat safe food and drink safe water when traveling in undeveloped areas. Use condoms, especially in anal sex. Food (especially shellfish) should be boiled for more than 90 s or heated to 85 °C for 4 min before eating. Contaminants should be disinfected by a 1:100 solution of household bleach. Avoid contact with uncooked foods when in the endemic area.

4.6.2.2.2 Institutions

The most effective ways are to improve environmental hygiene, provide safe food and water, and vaccinate hepatitis A vaccines. Hepatitis A transmission can be reduced by an adequate supply of safe water, proper treatment of sewage in the community, and promotion of personal hygiene practices.

4.6.2.2.3 Case Management

Patients with hepatitis A usually require only supportive care, such as rest when appropriate, adequate nutrition and hydration, avoidance of hepatotoxic agents such as alcohol and acetaminophen. Antiemetics may be used for severe vomiting, and antipyretics used for high fever. Renal function testing and blood analysis may be done to monitor kidney injury or hemolysis. No specific antiviral therapy is available for the treatment of the hepatitis A virus.

Hospitalization may be required in cases of complications, such as dehydration due to nausea and vomiting, severe prostration, liver failure which may be characterized by coagulopathy, encephalopathy, and/or worsening jaundice.

4.6.2.2.4 Outbreak Control

Determine high-risk groups (e.g., employees and students of childcare institutions), and whether to conduct emergency vaccination among them.

Provide health advice to patients, close contacts, and relevant institutions. Ensure adequate toilets and sanitation facilities.

Health measures for childcare institutions and schools should be strengthened in community outbreaks. Close contacts should be vaccinated.

4.6.3 Case of Hepatitis A Outbreak

Hepatitis A in the USA

1. Background

A national hepatitis A pandemic occurs about every 10 years in the USA. All children aged 12–23 months have been recommended to receive the hepatitis A vaccine since 2006, therefore, the number of hepatitis A has been decreasing.

Multistate outbreak of hepatitis A infections caused by pomegranate seeds from Turkey in 2013 [29]. 165 cases of hepatitis A were confirmed in 10 states: California, Arizona, Colorado, New Mexico, Hawaii, New Hampshire, New Jersey, Nevada, Utah, and Wisconsin. Ages ranged from 1 to 84 years, and 58% of cases were between 40 and 64 years. Eleven cases under 18 years were not previously vaccinated. Fifty-five percent of the cases were women. The major outbreak strain of hepatitis A virus belonged to genotype 1B in 117 cases in 9 states. This genotype was rarely found in the USA but circulates in North African and the Middle East. By combining information gained from Food and Drug Administration (FDA)'s traceback and trace forward investigations and Centers for Disease Control and Prevention (CDC)'s epidemiological investigation, it was found that the outbreak was related to frozen pomegranate seeds. Hepatitis A virus was insensitive to cold and could survive on the surface of frozen pomegranate seeds for 1 month. Suppliers have voluntarily recalled specific batches of frozen pomegranate seeds. Retailers proactively informed more than 250,000 customers by automated phones and more than 10,000 of them vaccinated.

Multistate outbreak of hepatitis A was linked to frozen strawberries in 2016 [24]. 143 cases with hepatitis A were reported from 9 states: Arkansas, California, Maryland, New York, North Carolina, Oregon, Virginia, West Virginia, and Wisconsin. 129 of them were reported to have eaten a smoothie from Tropical Smoothie Café. FDA reported that hepatitis A virus contamination was found in multiple samples of frozen strawberries. The suppliers and distributors recalled frozen strawberries. CDCs recommended post-exposure prophylaxis for unvaccinated people who had eaten recalled strawberries. Post-exposure prophylaxis recommended people between the ages of 1 and 40 years to receive the hepatitis A vaccine, and for those outside of this age range, receive hepatitis A virus-specific immunoglobulin.

An outbreak of hepatitis A in Hawaii was linked to raw scallops imported from the Philippines from June 12 to October 9, 2016 [30, 31]. A total of 292 laboratory-confirmed cases of hepatitis A were reported. Restaurants and retailers were prohibited to serve or sell scallops in the whole state. The residents were encouraged to be vaccinated against hepatitis A.

Hepatitis A virus outbreaks associated with drug use and homelessness in 2017 [32]. 1521 hepatitis A infections were reported in California, Kentucky, Michigan, and Utah, with 1019 (67%) male cases, 1073 (71%) hospitalizations, and 41 (3%) deaths. Coinfection with hepatitis B virus and hepatitis C virus are 42 cases and 341 cases, respectively. A total of 866 patients were reported to have used drugs, be homeless, or both. Eighty-one cases were men who had sex with men (MSM). Hepatitis A outbreaks shifted from point-source associated with contaminated food to a large community with person-to-person transmission. Control measures were applied by CDC and affected local and state health departments through health advisories, public health education, and vaccination clinics. Hepatitis A vaccine was administered in jails, emergency departments, syringe exchange programs, drug treatment facilities, and shelters for the homeless. A field investigation was conducted among the homeless for health publicity and vaccination.

Forty-five cases of hepatitis A among MSM were reported in New York from January to August 2017. One female case who self-reported having sexual contact with a bisexual male resident of a New Yorker was found in the outbreak. Fifteen cases were hospitalized, and three cases reported receipt of the hepatitis A vaccine. Nineteen cases had traveled domestically during their incubation period. Eight cases had traveled to western European countries with outbreaks of hepatitis A infection among MSM [33].

2. What Can We Learn from the Outbreaks?

Early laboratory testing can help identify the source of infection, take measures to control the consumption of contaminated food, and cut off the transmission routes.

The extremely poor public health status is an important risk factor for hepatitis A outbreaks. More outbreaks of hepatitis occur in areas of poor sanitation and insufficient public toilets, with many vagrants gathering.

Risk factors including the sharing of syringes among drug users and anal sex in MSM. They are not only easy to cause the spread of bloodborne diseases (hepatitis B, hepatitis C, HIV), but also may cause foodborne diseases (hepatitis B).

Patients infected with hepatitis A are mainly of low income, with low coverage of hepatitis A vaccination. As the number of vulnerable people increases when the homeless and drug users gather, if someone is infected with hepatitis A, it is easy to cause the spread of the disease.

3. What Are the Implications for Public Health Practice?

With the rapid economic development, improvement of people's living conditions, and public health facilities, the incidence of hepatitis A decreases in most countries. However, the epidemic of hepatitis A in the USA indicates that hepatitis A cases or outbreaks may occur in areas of low economic development, densely populated, and with insufficient water supply facilities.

With the globalization of food supply and the increased convenience of logistics, hepatitis A contaminated food can cause the outbreak in many areas. A national/regional foodborne disease laboratory surveillance network should be set up to share the results of pathogen testing in real-time and track the source of infections.

References

1. WHO. Poliomyelitis. https://www.who.int/en/news-room/fact-sheets/detail/poliomyelitis. 2019.
2. Greene SA, Ahmed J, Datta SD, et al. Progress toward polio eradication—worldwide, January 2017–March 2019. MMWR. 2019;68(20):458–62.
3. WHO. Poliomyelitis disease outbreak news. https://www.who.int/csr/don/archive/disease/poliomyelitis/en/. 2019.

4. WHO. Immunization, Vaccines and Biologicals. https://www.who.int/immunization/monitoring_surveillance/data/en/. 2019.
5. Global Polio Eradication Initiative. Key At-Risk Countries. http://polioeradication.org/where-we-work/key-at-risk-countries/. 2019.
6. National Health and Family Planning Commission. PRC, Poliomyelitis Diagnosis (WS 294-2016). 2016.
7. Luo HM, Zhang Y, Wang XQ, et al. Identification and control of a poliomyelitis outbreak in Xinjiang, China. N Engl J Med. 2013;369(21):1981–90.
8. Wenzhou Y, Wushouer F, Haibo W, et al. Experience and lessons learned from the investigation of and response to imported wild poliovirus causing local transmission in Xinjiang Uygur Autonomous Region in 2011. Chin J Vac Immuniz. 2013;19(04):361–4.
9. WHO. Standard operating procedures; Responding to a poliovirus event or outbreak version, vol. 3. Geneva: World Health Organization; 2018.
10. WHO. Measles. https://www.who.int/immunization/diseases/measles/en/. 2019.
11. WHO. Measles—Global situation. https://www.who.int/csr/don/26-november-2019-measles-global_situation/en/. 2019.
12. Chinese Center for Disease Control and Prevention. Knowledge of measles prevention and control. Aust Health Rev. 2017;2:63.
13. WHO. WHO recommended strategies for the prevention and control of communicable diseases. Geneva: WHO Press; 2001.
14. National Health Commission. PRC, Diagnosis of Epidemic Cerebrospinal Meningitis (WS 295-2019). 2019.
15. GBD. 2015 Disease and Injury Incidence and Prevalence Collaborators. Prevalence, Global, regional, and national incidence, prevalence, and years lived with disability for 310 diseases and injuries, 1990-2015: a systematic analysis for the Global Burden of Disease Study 2015. Lancet. 2016;388(10053):1545–602.
16. Epidemic meningitis control in countries of the. African meningitis belt, 2018. Wkly Epidemiol Rec. 2019;94(14/15):169–88.
17. Yoshikawa H, Ebihara K, Tanaka Y, et al. Efficacy of quadrivalent human papillomavirus (types 6, 11, 16 and 18) vaccine (GARDASIL) in Japanese women aged 18-26 years. Cancer Sci. 2013;104(4):465–72.
18. Ministry of Health, PRC. National Program for Epidemic Cerebrospinal Meningitis Prevention and Control (CDC [2006] No. 32). 2006.
19. Greenwood B. Manson lecture. Meningococcal meningitis in Africa. Trans R Soc Trop Med Hyg. 1999;93(4):341–53.
20. Yixing L, Junhong L, Zundong Y, et al. Surveillance and control of epidemic Japanese encephalitis. Chin J Plan Immuniz. 2006;6:527–32.
21. Fischer M, Lindsey N, Staples JE, et al. Japanese encephalitis vaccines: recommendations of the Advisory Committee on Immunization Practices (ACIP). MMWR. 2010;59(RR-1):1–27.
22. Instructions for the Prevention and Control of. Epidemic Japanese Encephalitis. Chin J Plan Immuniz. 2004;4:63–4.
23. Guoqiang W. Disease prevention and control in China 1955–2015. Beijing: China Population Publishing House; 2015.
24. Centers for Disease Control and Prevention. Yellow book 2020: health information for international travel. New York: Oxford University Press; 2017.
25. WHO. Hepatitis A. https://www.who.int/immunization/diseases/hepatitisA/en/. 2019.
26. Epidemiological update: hepatitis A outbreak in the EU/EEA mostly affecting men who have sex with men. https://www.ecdc.europa.eu/en/news-events/epidemiological-update-hepatitis-outbreak-eueea-mostly-affecting-men-who-have-sex-men-0. 2017.
27. Jacobsen KH, Wiersma ST. Hepatitis A virus seroprevalence by age and world region, 1990 and 2005. Vaccine. 2010;28(41):6653–7.
28. Fiore AE, Wasley A, Bell BP, et al. Prevention of hepatitis A through active or passive immunization: recommendations of the Advisory Committee on Immunization Practices (ACIP). MMWR. 2006;55(Rr-7):1–23.

29. Collier MG, Khudyakov YE, Selvage D, et al. Outbreak of hepatitis A in the USA associated with frozen pomegranate arils imported from Turkey: an epidemiological case study. Lancet Infect Dis. 2014;14(10):976–81.
30. State of Hawaii, Department of Health. Hepatitis A Outbreak 2016. http://health.hawaii.gov/docd/hepatitis-a-outbreak-2016/. 2016.
31. CDC. Outbreak of hepatitis A in Hawaii linked to raw scallops. https://www.cdc.gov/hepatitis/outbreaks/2016/hav-hawaii.htm. 2016.
32. Foster M, Ramachandran S, Myatt K, et al. Hepatitis A virus outbreaks associated with drug use and homelessness—California, Kentucky, Michigan, and Utah, 2017. MMWR. 2018;67(43):1208–10.
33. Latash J, Dorsinville M, Del Rosso P, et al. Notes from the field: increase in reported hepatitis A infections among men who have sex with men—New York City, January–August 2017. MMWR. 2017;66(37):999–1000.

Risks of Tuberculosis Prevention and Control

5

Caihong Xu and Hui Zhang

Tuberculosis (TB) is a chronic infectious disease caused by *Mycobacterium tuberculosis*, which is seriously harmful to human health. *Mycobacterium tuberculosis* mainly affects the human lungs, resulting in pulmonary tuberculosis and even extrapulmonary tuberculosis. *Mycobacterium tuberculosis* can be transmitted by air, and people are mainly infected via droplets produced by patients who discharge the bacteria while speaking loudly or coughing. People are generally susceptible to infection.

5.1 Epidemic Situation of Tuberculosis

Since the beginning of the twentieth century, the prevalence of TB has been effectively controlled in many countries. In the late 1980s, however, many developed and developing countries witnessed the return of the TB epidemic. As a result, the WHO had to declare "a global TB emergency" in 1993. So far, the incidence of TB in many countries remains high, and outbreaks occur in some areas from time to time. The problem of drug resistance and the transmission of *Mycobacterium tuberculosis* is also a serious challenge worldwide.

5.1.1 General Situation of Global TB

In 2016, WHO announced the list of 30 countries with high burden of TB, TB/HIV coinfection, and MDR-TB in 2016–2020, including (bold county names mean high burden of TB, MDR-TB, and TB/HIV coinfection) **Angola**, Bangladesh, Brazil,

C. Xu · H. Zhang (✉)
Chinese Center for Disease Control and Prevention, Beijing, People's Republic of China
e-mail: zhanghui@chinacdc.cn

W. Yang (ed.), *Prevention and Control of Infectious Diseases in BRI Countries*,
https://doi.org/10.1007/978-981-33-6958-0_5

Cambodia, **China**, Congo, Central Africa, Democratic People's Republic of Korea, the **Democratic Republic of the Congo**, **Ethiopia, India, Indonesia, Kenya**, Lesotho, Liberia, **Mozambique, Burma**, Namibia, **Nigeria**, Pakistan, Papua New Guinea, Philippines, Russia, Sierra Leone, South Africa, Thailand, **Tanzania**, Vietnam, Zambia, and **Zimbabwe**.

1. New TB cases: Globally, it was estimated that around 10 million people developed TB disease in 2017, with an incidence of 133/100,000, including 6.36 million men, 3.68 million women, and 1.01 million children [1]. In 2017, it was estimated that most of the cases occurred in the WHO Southeast Asian region (44%), African region (25%), and the Western Pacific region (18%), while a small number occurred in the eastern Mediterranean region (7.7%), the American region (2.8%), and the European region (2.7%). Thirty high TB burden countries accounted for 87.2% of the world's cases, and two-thirds were in eight countries: India (27%), China (9%), Indonesia (8%), the Philippines (6%), Pakistan (5%), Nigeria (4%), Bangladesh (4%), and South Africa (3%).
2. New MDR/RR-TB cases: It was estimated that worldwide in 2017, 560,000 people developed TB that was resistant to multiple drugs/rifampicin (MDR/RR), and of these, around 82% had multidrug-resistant TB (MDR-TB). 3.6% of new TB cases and 17.0% of previously treated cases had RR-TB. The number of new RR-TB cases in these 30 countries was about 507,000, accounting for 90.5% of the global total. Three countries accounted for about 47% of the world's cases of MDR/RR-TB: India, China, and the Russian Federation (10%).
3. New TB/HIV coinfections: In 2017, 920,000 of the estimated 10 million TB patients in the world were HIV positive, accounting for about 9%, and the incidence was 9.2/100,000. Among them, 766,000 TB/HIV coinfections were in high burden countries, accounting for 83% of the global total.
4. TB deaths and mortality: It was estimated that in 2017, about 1.57 million people died of TB in the world, with a mortality rate of 17/100,000. The ranking of TB as the leading causes of death has changed from the 9th to the 10th, but it is still one of the top 10 causes of death in the world. Among the 30 countries, the largest number of TB deaths is in India (410,000) and the lowest is in Namibia (8000), while the highest TB mortality is in Mozambique (73/100,000) and the lowest is in Brazil (2.4/100,000).

5.1.2 TB Epidemic in the "Belt and Road" Countries

Among the "Belt and Road" countries, 12 countries (India, Indonesia, Bangladesh, Pakistan, Cambodia, Burma, Philippines, Thailand, Vietnam, Ethiopia, Kenya, and Russia) were among those with high burden of TB in 2016–2020 announced by WHO, while 13 countries or province (India, Russia, Ukraine, Pakistan, Philippines, Burma, Uzbekistan, Indonesia, Vietnam, Kazakhstan, Bangladesh, Kenya, and Thailand) were among those with high burden of MDR-TB in 2016–2020 announced by WHO (Table 5.1).

Table 5.1 TB epidemic in countries along the "Belt and Road"

	TB cases (10,000)	Incidence (/100,000)	TB/HIV coinfections (10,000)	MDR/RR cases (10,000)	Deaths (10,000)	Mortality rate (/100,000)
India	274	204/10	8.6	13.5	41	31/10
Indonesia	84.2	319/10	3.6	2.3	10.7	40/10
Bangladesh	36.4	221/10	0.055	0.84	5.9	36/10
Pakistan	52.5	267/10	0.73	2.7	5.4	27/10
Cambodia	5.2	326/10	0.13	0.12	0.31	19/10
Burma	19.1	358/10	1.7	1.4	2.7	51/10
Philippines	58.1	554/10	0.71	2.7	2.6	25/10
Thailand	10.8	156/10	1.1	0.39	0.93	13/10
Vietnam	12.4	129/10	0.45	0.71	1.2	12/10
Ethiopia	17.2	164/10	1.2	0.55	2.5	24/10
Kenya	15.8	319/10	4.5	0.28	2.5	50/10
Russia	8.6	60/10	1.8	5.6	1	7.3/10

5.1.3 TB Epidemic in China

The number of reported TB patients in China in 2017 was 835,000, ranking the second in category A and B infectious diseases in China. The reported incidence of TB is decreasing year by year, from 74.3/100,000 in 2010 to 60.5/100,000 in 2017, or an annual decline rate of 3.2% higher than that globally (1.5%).

Globally, China's TB burden is second only to India. WHO estimated that in 2017, new TB cases in China totaled 889,000, or 8.9% of the global total, and 49.4% that of the Western Pacific region. The estimated TB incidence in 2017 was 63/100,000, ranking 28th among the 30 countries with high TB burden.

In 2017, 12,000 TB/HIV coinfections were estimated in China, ranking 14th among the 30 countries, and the incidence, 0.8/100,000, or 27th among the 30 countries.

The RR-TB rates of new cases and retreated cases in China were 7.1% and 24.0%, respectively. According to the estimated cases of TB, the number of RR-TB cases was 73,000 (13% of, or second in the global total); the number of RR-TB cases calculated according to the number of identified TB patients was 58,000; the number of RR-TB cases calculated according to the number of identified smear-positive TB patients was 21,000.

TB deaths in China was 37,000, and the death rate, 2.6/100,000, ranking the 29th among the 30 countries [2].

5.2 TB Risks and Principles for Prevention and Control

5.2.1 TB Prevention and Control Strategy in "Belt and Road" Countries

The strategy of Directly Observed Therapy (DOTS) was developed by Karel Styblo from the International Union against TB and Lung Disease in the 1970s and 1980s. It consists of five elements: government commitment, case detection by sputum smear microscopy, standardized treatment regimens directly observed for smear-positive TB patients, regular and uninterrupted supply of free anti-TB drugs, and standardized recording, reporting, surveillance, and assessment system for TB patients. According to years of experience in piloting and replication around the world, the DOTS strategy can identify the source of infection to the greatest extent and can cure almost all newly identified TB patients. Patients do not need to be hospitalized, and the cost of treatment is low. In 1994, WHO announced that the DOTS strategy is the most cost-effective way to stop the spread of TB and recommended it as a global TB control strategy.

In March 2006, WHO and the Stop TB Partnership proposed a new TB control strategy in order to actively respond to the MDR-TB and TB/HIV coinfection and achieve the Millennium Development Goals of the United Nations. The core of the strategy is DOTS, and it also complements and improves the implementation of the DOTS strategy, its fairness and quality, so as to ensure that all TB patients can obtain diagnosis and treatment. Its six components include to (1) expand and enhance quality DOTS; (2) focus on challenges of TB/HIV comorbidity and multidrug-resistant TB (MDR-TB, for instance); (3) strengthen primary health care; (4) engage all care providers; (5) encourage people with TB; (6) strengthen and promote scientific research.

The "End TB Strategy" was adopted at the 67th World Health Assembly in 2014 [3]. The VISION of the Strategy is a world free of TB—zero deaths, disease, and sufferings due to TB. The GOAL is to end the global TB epidemic by 2035 (TB incidence <10/100,000), a 95% reduction in TB deaths (compared with 2015), and no affected families facing catastrophic costs due to TB. Meanwhile, in order to better achieve the goal of ending TB by 2035, the strategy also sets the interim goals for 2020 and 2025: 20% reduction in TB incidence rate and 35% reduction in TB deaths (compared with 2015) globally, or incidence rate <85/100,000 by 2020, and 50% reduction in TB incidence rate and 75% reduction in TB deaths (compared with 2015) globally, or incidence rate <50/100,000 by 2025. At its core, there are three pillars: integrated, patient-centered care and prevention; bold policies and supportive systems; and intensified research and innovation. To actively respond to the "End TB Strategy," the Chinese government issued the "13th Five-Year Plan for Tuberculosis Prevention and Control" in 2017, which clearly states that "By 2020, the incidence of pulmonary TB throughout China shall be reduced to 58/100,000." The "Outline of 'Healthy China 2030' Program" (hereinafter referred to as the

Outline) puts forward an explicit plan for the TB control system, that is, "to establish a model for integrated TB prevention and care services, to strengthen the screening and surveillance of MDR-TB, to standardize TB diagnosis, treatment and management, and to ensure the continued reduction in TB epidemic throughout the country." The Outline also points out that by 2030, the proportion of personal health expenses in total health expenditure shall be reduced to less than 25%, and the universal health coverage shall be achieved. Based on this goal, public financing is expected to increase to raise the level of medical insurance, and in turn, to reduce the economic burden for patients.

5.2.2 Risk of the Spread of TB Epidemic from Other "Belt and Road" Countries to China, and Recommendations on Its Prevention and Control

India, Indonesia, Bangladesh, Pakistan, Cambodia, Burma, Philippines, Thailand, Vietnam, Ethiopia, Kenya, Russia, Ukraine, Uzbekistan, and Kazakhstan are among the 30 countries with high burden of TB and/or MDR-TB in 2016–2020 announced by WHO. There is a risk of the import of TB, particularly MDR-TB, from these countries to China. If foreign TB patients, particularly MDR-TB patients, stay in China for a long period of time, the transmission risk will increase. If they stay in hospitals, prisons, schools, and other congregation settings for a long period of time, and adequate infection control measures are not taken, it may cause local transmission.

China needs to establish a joint prevention and control mechanism for infectious diseases with the above countries. According to recommendations in "Tuberculosis and Air Travel" published by WHO, the "Belt and Road" countries are required to restrict TB patients, especially those with MDR-TB, to make international travel during the infectious period. It prohibits patients with known infectious TB to take public aircraft before they are adequately treated for at least 2 weeks or MDR-TB patients to travel before they are fully tested (i.e., culture) and proved noninfectious. To avoid local spread caused by the import of TB into China, relevant provisions of the Law of the People's Republic of China on the Administration of Exit and Entry provide that no visa shall be issued to patients with infectious TB. If patients with infectious TB or MDR-TB are found to travel internationally, the countries concerned shall inform each other so that the target country can take preventive and control measures in time and reduce the risk of local transmission.

Once there are TB cases imported from abroad, the CDC shall actively strengthen the surveillance, track cases, assist designated health facilities to carry out appropriate TB treatment and management, take the initiative to contact the close contacts of the infectious TB patients for testing according to relevant provisions, and take effective follow-up actions.

5.2.3 Risk for Travelling to and Working in "Belt and Road" Countries, and Recommendations on Travel

Although travel and work-related risks of TB infection are lower in most "Belt and Road" countries than in China, it is recommended that travelers stay away from high-risk settings, such as crowded hospitals, prisons, and homeless shelters. If they need to visit such places, they are recommended to wear masks.

The common symptoms of TB include discomfort or weakness, weight loss, fever, and night sweat. There may also be cough, chest pain, and hemoptysis. Other symptoms of extrapulmonary TB are related to the affected parts. Individuals with the above symptoms should stop their international travels, as are recommended in "Tuberculosis and Air Travel" published by WHO. Patients with known infectious TB shall not take public aircraft before they are adequately treated for at least 2 weeks. MDR-TB patients shall not travel until they have been fully tested (i.e., culture) and proved in a noninfectious status. If the patients have left the country, they should contact local physicians or health departments for active treatment, prevention, and control [4–7].

5.2.4 Recommendations on Public Health Cooperation Among "Belt and Road" Countries

In consideration of the development level of the public health and the epidemic patterns of TB in "Belt and Road" countries, China can cooperate with "Belt and Road" countries in joint prevention and control of TB, especially MDR-TB and TB/HIV coinfection, public health system strengthening, professional communication and training, scientific research, etc.

5.3 Case Studies on Prevention and Control

Case 1: A Typical Case of Investigation and Control of Tuberculosis Outbreak in School

1. Outbreak identification: On March 11, 2016, a student in a university was diagnosed as a sputum smear-positive pulmonary TB case and was notified in the National Disease Surveillance Information Management System. The local Center for Disease Control and Prevention (CDC) interviewed the student and discovered that he had been coughing since December 2015 and had already been diagnosed as a TB case in January 2016 in his hometown during his winter holiday. The student returned to the university after the holiday and purposely concealed his disease.

The CDC immediately organized a close contact investigation on March 11th and screened all 80 students who were in the same class and the same dormitory with this TB case. Two new TB cases were diagnosed, and 17 students strongly positive in tuberculin susceptibility test (TST) (indicated TB infection) were identified. Since new cases were discovered, a series of screenings and outbreak surveys were carried out in this university on more students and teachers who might have contacted those TB cases closely or casually. Finally, from March 11th to 30th, 424 students and teachers were screened with chest X-ray examination and TST, and 12 pulmonary tuberculosis cases were diagnosed. Thus, based on the identified epidemiological linkage from a detailed analysis of investigation information, this outbreak was reported as a public health emergency to local health authorities.

2. Emergency responses: The local government took rapid actions to respond to this public health emergency, including (1) investigating and screening all related persons to figure out new cases and identify disease spreading route; (2) isolating all diagnosed TB cases, enhancing treatment supervision for 1 inpatient and 11 outpatients isolated at home or school; (3) The prescribing preventive therapy for 28 (of the 41) TST strongly positive students without TB) agreed to take preventive treatment; (4) enhancing ventilation in all classrooms and dormitories, conducting air sterilization in places where those TB cases stayed; (5) organizing health education activities among students and teachers to inform them of early symptoms of TB and how to protect themselves, hence dispelling their fears for TB; (6) intensifying TB symptom monitoring and reporting in schools for early detection and reference of students with suspected symptoms to TB designated hospitals; (7) soothing emotions of TB cases and their parents and making plans to help students catch up with their courses even if they had to leave school for 4–6 months for anti-TB treatment; (8) releasing newsletters about this emergency event and communicating with medias to inform the society promptly of the progress of the emergency response.

The investigation showed that 9 TB cases lived on the same floor of a dormitory building, two lived on the upper floor of this building, and one lived in another building but shared the classroom with one case. Thus, it was believed that the outbreak was mainly due to TB spreading in dormitories. Since the last case being detected through screening on March 24th, no new case was found. All diagnosed cases finished anti-TB treatment and were cured in 6 months. The local government ended emergency response 3 months after the last case was diagnosed.

3. Lessons learned: First, school TB prevention and control measures were not well implemented. Otherwise, the index case should have been found to be a suspected TB case and reported and referred to the local TB hospital to shorten the time of disease spreading in school. Second, the TB hospital in the index case's hometown should have verified the case's occupation and notified him as a student so that the information could be transferred to the CDC of the county where the university is located. Third, preventive therapy is an important measure for preventing infected students from developing into active TB cases. We should try to persuade as many as possible of those infected students to take preventive treatment. Finally, the excellent collaboration of health and education departments should always be the essential foundation for rapid response to public health emergencies.

References

1. World Health Organization. Global tuberculosis report, 2018. Geneva, Switzerland: WHO; 2018.
2. China CDC. Chinese Annual Report on TB Surveillance of 2018.
3. Lonnroth K, Raviglione M. WHO's new "End TB Strategy" in the post-2015 era of the sustainable development goals. Trans R Soc Trop Med Hyg. 2016;110:148–50. https://doi.org/10.1093/trstmh/trv108.
4. Seaworth BJ, Armitige LY, Aronson NE, et al. Multidrug-resistant tuberculosis. Recommendations for reducing risk during travel for healthcare and humanitarian work. Ann Am Thorac Soc. 2014;11(3):286–95. https://doi.org/10.1513/AnnalsATS.201309-312PS.
5. Martinez L, Blanc L, Nunn P, et al. Tuberculosis and air travel: WHO guidance in the era of drug-resistant TB. Travel Med Infect Dis. 2008;6(4):177–81. https://doi.org/10.1016/j.tmaid.2007.10.004.
6. Martinez L, Thomas K, Figueroa J. Guidance from WHO on the prevention and control of TB during air travel. Travel Med Infect Dis. 2010;8(2):84–9. https://doi.org/10.1016/j.tmaid.2009.02.005.
7. Plotkin BJ, Hardiman MC. The international health regulations (2005), tuberculosis and air travel. Travel Med Infect Dis. 2010;8(2):90–5. https://doi.org/10.1016/j.tmaid.2009.11.003.

The Risk and Prevention and Control of Influenza

6

Jiandong Zheng and Luzhao Feng

Influenza is a contagious respiratory illness caused by influenza viruses that infect the nose, throat, and sometimes the lungs. It can cause mild-to-severe illness, and at times, deaths. According to core proteins and matrix proteins, the influenza viruses can be divided into four types: A, B, C, and D. Human influenza A and B viruses cause a seasonal epidemic of disease around the world every year. A pandemic can occur when a new and very different influenza A virus that can infect people and spread fast between people emerges. Influenza type C infections generally cause mild illness and are not thought to cause human flu epidemics. Influenza D viruses primarily affect cattle, and it is not sure whether they can infect or cause illness in people.

Influenza A viruses are divided into subtypes based on two proteins on the surface of the virus: hemagglutinin (H) and neuraminidase (N). There are 18 different hemagglutinin subtypes and 11 different neuraminidase subtypes (H1 to H18 and N1 to N11, respectively). Therefore, there are potentially 198 different influenza A subtype combinations. Influenza A (H1N1 and H3N2) viruses cause seasonal epidemics in humans every year. In the spring of 2009, a new type of influenza A (H1N1) virus emerged and caused the first influenza pandemic in the twenty-first century, more than 40 years after the Hong Kong influenza pandemic in 1968. This new type of virus subsequently replaced the seasonal influenza A (H1N1) virus circulated before 2009. Influenza B viruses are not divided into subtypes, but instead, further classified into two lineages: B/Yamagata and B/Victoria.

The original version of this chapter was revised. A correction to this chapter is available at https://doi.org/10.1007/978-981-33-6958-0_15

J. Zheng
Chinese Center for Disease Control and Prevention, Beijing, People's Republic of China

L. Feng (✉)
Chinese Academy of Medical Sciences & Peking Union Medical College, Beijing, People's Republic of China
e-mail: fengluzhao@cams.cn

W. Yang (ed.), *Prevention and Control of Infectious Diseases in BRI Countries*, https://doi.org/10.1007/978-981-33-6958-0_6

Influenza A viruses with low genetic stability and prone to mutation and reassortment are found in many different animals, such as ducks, chickens, pigs, horses, cats, and dogs. Genetic mutation is the cause of changes in the subtype and strains of the human seasonal influenza viruses, and also the biological basis for cross-species transmission of zoonotic influenza viruses. The spread of influenza A virus among animals, especially chickens, frequently causes substantial losses to the poultry industry. Zoonotic influenza A virus can occasionally spread across species, infecting people or causing illness in them. For example, there has been human infection with avian influenza H5N1, H7N9, H5N6, and H10N8 viruses since 2003 in China, and the case fatality rate of H5N1 and H5N6 has reached 60%. Fortunately, these avian influenza viruses cannot spread easily among humans. Influenza A viruses from different species could infect the same person or animal, mix existing genetic information (reassortment), and produce a new influenza A virus. If this virus with genetic reassortment could infect people easily and spread from person to person in an efficient and sustained way, it is likely to cause a new influenza pandemic that spread quickly across the world. Further, the number of patients, hospitalizations, and deaths can be significantly higher in an influenza pandemic than in seasonal influenza, and social and economic activities were seriously impacted, hence huge damages to human health and the economy. In 1918–1919, the number of deaths in the Spanish pandemic caused by an H1N1 virus with genes of avian origin was estimated to be at least 50 million worldwide. It was the most serious disaster of medical science in the twentieth century.

6.1 Overview of the Influenza/Avian Influenza Epidemic in "Belt and Road" ("B&R") Countries

Influenza was the first disease to be monitored globally. Global influenza surveillance has been conducted through WHO's Global Influenza Surveillance and Response System (GISRS) since 1952. The mission of GISRS is to protect people from the threat of influenza by constantly recommending vaccine strains for annual seasonal influenza vaccine production, vaccine prototype strains with potential pandemic risk in response to influenza pandemics. Another mission of GISRS is continuously updating influenza virus detection and surveillance reagents based on global surveillance data, providing the scientific basis for clinical antiviral treatment through monitoring drug resistance, ongoing risk assessment for influenza epidemic and pandemic.

6.1.1 Seasonal Influenza

The influenza intensity and dominant strains vary with climates and areas (Fig. 6.1 [1]). In the temperate zone, seasonal epidemics occur mainly in winter and spring each year. In tropical regions, influenza activity shows a highly diverse

Number of specimens positive for influenza

Northern hemisphere

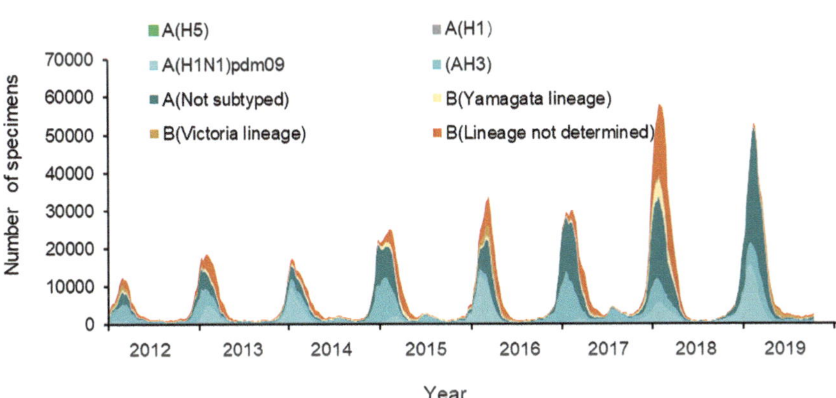

Southern hemisphere

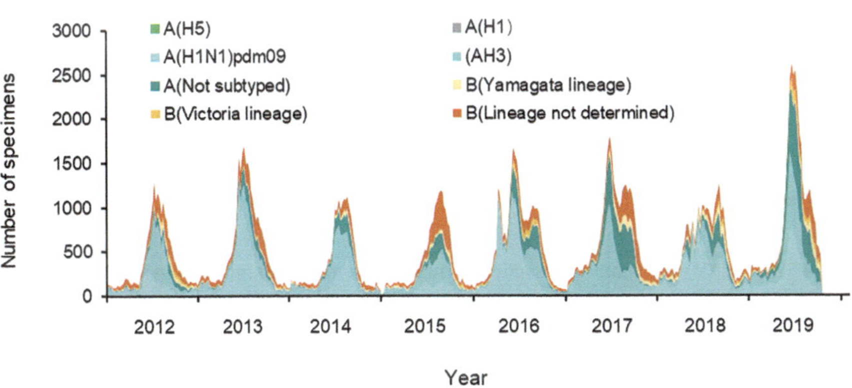

Fig. 6.1 Number of specimens positive for influenza by subtype in the Northern and Southern hemisphere from the 1st week of 2012 to the 40th week of 2019

seasonal pattern, which can be cyclically endemic for 6 months (summer peak) or throughout the whole year, causing outbreaks more irregularly. Take influenza surveillance data as of October 25, 2019 as example, in the northern "B&R" including China, Mongolia, Russia, and several countries in Central Asia, the dominant strain was influenza A(H3N2) and the influenza activity was extremely low or inactive while there were influenza A (H3N2), influenza A (H1N1), and dominant influenza B viruses co-circulated with much higher positive rate of influenza virus in the southern "B&R".

6.1.2 Avian Influenza

Avian influenza refers to the disease caused by infection with avian influenza type A viruses. These viruses exist naturally among wild aquatic birds worldwide and can infect domestic poultry and other bird and animal species. Sporadic human infections with avian flu viruses have occurred. Avian influenza viruses cannot spread easily from person to person. Avian influenza can cause mild-to-severe illness, including death. An outbreak of highly pathogenic avian influenza A (H5N1) caused 18 infections and 6 deaths in Hong Kong in 1997. Since 2003, H5N1 and other avian influenza viruses have spread from Asia to Europe and Africa. In 2013, China reported the first case of human infection with avian influenza A (H7N9) virus. It experienced several waves of the epidemic and the cases totaled over one thousand, among which only three were reported abroad and all of them were epidemiologically related to China. As of September 2019, a total of 861 cases of A (H5N1), including 455 deaths, had been identified in 17 countries around the world, most of which were in "B&R" countries in South Asia, Southeast Asia, and Egypt (Table 6.1 [2]). Since the first case of avian influenza A (H5N6) reported in Sichuan province in April 2014, a total of 24 cases of H5N6 avian influenza have been reported in China Mainland, with 16 deaths, or fatality rate, 66.7%.

With current scientific knowledge and technology, it is impossible to predict when and where such a pandemic will occur, the virus strain that causes it, and how serious it will be (as mild as the pandemic A (H1N1) 2009, or as catastrophic as the 1918 Spanish pandemic), but it will definitely happen in the future. Due to economic globalization, urbanization, and increasing mobility, not only "B&R" countries but also various regions of the world will be affected severely within 1 or 2 months if influenza pandemic occurs.

Table 6.1 Cumulative number of confirmed human case for avian influenza A (H5N1) reported to WHO, 2003–2019

Country	2003-2009*		2010-2014*		2015		2016		2017		2018		2019		Total	
	cases	deaths	cases	deaths	cases	deaths	cases	deaths	cases	deaths	cases	deaths	cases	deaths	cases	deaths
Azerbaijan	8	5	0	0	0	0	0	0	0	0	0	0	0	0	8	5
Bangladesh	1	0	6	1	1	0	0	0	0	0	0	0	0	0	8	1
Cambodia	9	7	47	30	0	0	0	0	0	0	0	0	0	0	56	37
Canada	0	0	1	1	0	0	0	0	0	0	0	0	0	0	1	1
China	38	25	9	5	6	1	0	0	0	0	0	0	0	0	53	31
Djibouti	1	0	0	0	0	0	0	0	0	0	0	0	0	0	1	0
Egypt	90	27	120	50	136	39	10	3	3	1	0	0	0	0	359	120
Indonesia	162	134	35	31	2	2	0	0	1	1	0	0	0	0	200	168
Iraq	3	2	0	0	0	0	0	0	0	0	0	0	0	0	3	2
Lao People's Democratic Republic	2	2	0	0	0	0	0	0	0	0	0	0	0	0	2	2
Myanmar	1	0	0	0	0	0	0	0	0	0	0	0	0	0	1	0
Nepal	0	0	0	0	0	0	0	0	0	0	0	0	1	1	1	1
Nigeria	1	1	0	0	0	0	0	0	0	0	0	0	0	0	1	1
Pakistan	3	1	0	0	0	0	0	0	0	0	0	0	0	0	3	1
Thailand	25	17	0	0	0	0	0	0	0	0	0	0	0	0	25	17
Turkey	12	4	0	0	0	0	0	0	0	0	0	0	0	0	12	4
Viet Nam	112	57	15	7	0	0	0	0	0	0	0	0	0	0	127	64
Total	468	282	233	125	145	42	10	3	4	2	0	0	1	1	861	455

* 2003-2009 total figures. Breakdowns by year available on subsequent tables.
** 2010-2014 total figures. Breakdowns by year available on subsequent tables.
Total nuber of cases includes number of dearhs
WHO reports only laboratory cases.
All dated refer to onset of illness.
Source: WHO/GIP, data in HQ as of 27 September 2019

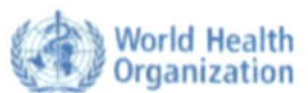

6.2 The Risk and Principles for the Prevention and Control of Influenza

6.2.1 The Risk of Epidemic

Annual influenza vaccination is the most cost-effective way to prevent seasonal influenza. However, influenza vaccines can only provide moderate protection if the circulating influenza viruses are well-matched to the flu vaccine. Although the national influenza vaccination rate in the United States is close to 50% [3], influenza still causes a large number of illnesses, hospitalizations and deaths every year. Depending on its intensity and severity, it can affect tens of millions of people and causes tens of thousands or even 60,000 deaths in US [4]. "B&R" countries will inevitably have influenza epidemics in winter, spring, and summer or throughout the year, as may vary to their climatic zones.

The US CDC uses the Influenza Risk Assessment Tool (IRAT) to assess 16 new subtypes of influenza A viruses, including H7N9. The H7N9 virus was found to have the highest risk score and was characterized as having a medium to high risk of a potential pandemic [5]. Surveillance data in China found that despite the highly pathogenic H7N9 virus in poultry outbreaks and human infections, there were no significant changes in its etiology, main infection routes, and patterns of cases. The H7N9 virus is still of bird origin, and its route of infection is still from bird to human. Contact with infected birds or exposure to live poultry markets are still important risk factors for human infection. In view of the wide distribution of H7, H5, and H9 viruses in poultry and the environment, and the basically unchanged pattern of poultry farming, transportation, and consumption, human infection with existing avian influenza viruses will continue in the future. There is also the possibility of cases of infection with new subtype influenza viruses. However, the scale of poultry and human epidemics will remain within controllable range. China has implemented a lot of stringent live poultry market management measures, stressed cross-regional transport management of live poultry, and provided (by the Ministry of Agriculture) compulsory immunization of poultry throughout the country in recent years. As the family poultry production patterns and consumption habits of live poultry in some "B&R" countries are similar to those in China, the possibility of local cases infected with the avian influenza virus cannot be ruled out. As long as the infection of humans with animal-derived influenza continues, a pandemic influenza virus may appear at any time.

6.2.2 Prevention and Control Principles

6.2.2.1 Seasonal Influenza

In summary, China has been persistent in "enhancing surveillance and early warning, immunizing high-risk populations, regulating epidemic management, implementing medical treatment, and conducting extensive publicity and mobilization."

Surveillance is the foundation of prevention and control for all diseases. Influenza vaccination is the most effective way to prevent influenza. People above 6 months of age and without contraindications can be vaccinated. Children aged 6 months through 4 years (59 months), the elderly, people with underlying conditions, pregnant women, and medical staff are the priority population to be recommended for vaccination. Clusters and outbreaks of influenza are unavoidable, and they need to be controlled timely to curb the spread of the epidemic once detected. Scientific diagnosis and treatment of influenza cases can not only prevent the emergence of resistant strains but also shorten the course of the disease and reduce the occurrence of severe cases and deaths. Through publicity and mobilization, comprehensive prevention and control of influenza could be carried out by improving people's awareness of influenza and vaccines, advocating healthy lifestyles, developing good hygiene practices, and adopting nonpharmaceutic interventions (NPIs). NPIs usually include avoiding close contact, staying at home when being sick, covering your mouth and nose with a tissue when coughing or sneezing, cleaning hands, avoiding touching your eyes, nose or mouth, etc.

6.2.2.2 Avian Influenza

After assessing China's response to the avian influenza H7N9 epidemic in 2013, WHO stated that "China's response to the H7N9 avian influenza epidemic is a global model."

A series of scientific research carried out after the outbreak has timely identified the key epidemiological characteristics of the disease, and has provided scientific evidence for H7N9 epidemic prevention strategies and measures, which, with the involving understanding of the disease and judgment of the epidemic situation, were timely adjusted at different stages of the epidemic. This was of great significance for stabilizing society, avoiding panic, and ensuring national security while reducing economic losses. The specific measures were as following:

- Disease surveillance and risk assessment: carry out surveillance on cases, the environment, and live poultry and conduct epidemic detection, risk assessment, early warning, etc.
- Reduce the risk of human exposure and infection: suspend live poultry trading, close live poultry markets, etc.
- Control outbreaks in poultry: vaccinate poultry, cull infected poultry, manage the cross-regional transport of live poultry, etc.
- Patients' clinical treatment and medical management: timely release and update case diagnosis and treatment plan of human avian influenza A (H7N9) cases and adopt "four concentration" and "four early" principles, that is, "concentration of patients, experts, resources, and treatment" and "early detection, reporting, diagnosis, and treatment."
- Communicate risks and public opinion guidance: disseminate authoritative and scientific epidemic information to the public in a targeted manner, publicize knowledge of prevention and control, and respond to social concerns in a timely manner.

6.3 Cases of Influenza Prevention and Control

The Response to Pandemic A (H1N1) 2009 in China

1. Overview

Since the twentieth century, there have been four pandemics worldwide, the most serious of which was the Spanish flu of 1918, which killed about 20–50 million people worldwide [6]. Almost a century after it, the pandemic H1N1 2009 influenza virus began to spread from Mexico and the United States to the whole world. As of August 1, 2010, laboratory-confirmed influenza A (H1N1) cases had been reported in more than 214 countries and regions, including at least 18,449 deaths [7]. It was estimated that the number of respiratory and cardiovascular deaths due to influenza A (H1N1) infection was more than 15 times the number reported [8].

The first human case of H1N1 in China was an imported case from the United States, discovered by the Chengdu Center for Disease Control (Chengdu CDC), and then confirmed by Sichuan Center for Disease Control (Sichuan CDC) and the Chinese Center for Disease Control and Prevention (China CDC). Within a short period, local cases also appeared one after another, and the epidemic spread rapidly to all provinces and cities nationwide. According to a nationwide cross-sectional seroprevalence study [9], an estimated number of 200 million individuals (16%) were infected with H1N1 in China.

2. Strategies and Measures of Prevention and Control

When WHO announced that A (HINI) outbreak was an "international public health concern" on April 25, 2009, the emergency response actions were triggered immediately in China. Under the leadership of the State Council, a joint emergency response mechanism was timely established. In order to protect the public from security threats and to guarantee normal economic activities and social stability, all ministries were involved in a coordinated manner to fight against the A (HINI) pandemic.

2.1 Develop a Scientific-Based Strategy with a Timely Update to Different Epidemic Situations

After the SARS outbreak in 2003 and H5N1 human infection reported in 2005, China developed a pandemic response plan that covered surveillance, laboratory capacity building, vaccine development, and stockpiling.

To strictly prevent the imported case before the first confirmed human case was reported, it strengthened the exit–entry inspection and quarantine, enhanced surveillance, conducted communication and education campaigns, and carried out research on diagnostic reagents, antiviral drugs, and vaccines. After reporting the first case of human infection, the surveillance network was expanded and specific hospitals were designated to treat patients. After the pandemic was announced on June 11, 2009, the strategy was adjusted to strengthen prevention and control in schools and communities and to speed up clinical trials of vaccines. As the epidemic spread further, the strategy was adjusted again to improve clinical treatment and, in particular, to promote vaccination of severe cases and high-risk populations and strengthen risk communication and health promotion to reduce the impact of the epidemic and minimize its morbidity and mortality.

2.2 Develop Test Kit and Build Laboratory Surveillance Capacity

Chinese National Influenza Center (CNIC) developed the test kits successfully within 72 h after the US CDC provided the pandemic H1N1 virus and sequences. The test kits were distributed to all national influenza surveillance networks, quarantine and inspection laboratories, and other 13 countries, including Cuba and Mongolia. The influenza surveillance network was expanded from 63 laboratories to 411 laboratories in order to strengthen the diagnostic capacity in China.

2.3 Promote Vaccine Development and Vaccination Campaign

The pandemic influenza virus antigenicity is significantly different from seasonal H1N1, and the original trivalent seasonal influenza vaccines could not provide cross-protection. Therefore, relevant national ministries and ten influenza vaccine manufacturers have actively participated in vaccine development trials only 1 month after the pandemic was announced [10]. Eventually, the vaccine was approved for use in early September, making China the first country in the world to successfully complete vaccine development and registration.

2.4 Improve the Treatment of Patients

Clinical treatment in the healthcare system, with enhanced surgical capacity, is one of the most important components to mitigate the pandemic's impact. Clinical case management and treatment guidelines were rapidly developed and timely updated in China, and all confirmed patients received antiviral treatment in designated hospitals. Antivirals were also provided to close contacts at high risk for severe influenza. High-risk populations included pregnant women, those with chronic illnesses, children aged under 5 years, elders aged 65 and above, and healthcare workers. In addition, the Chinese government strengthened the treatment capacity of low-income provinces through additional investments in medical facilities and stockpiles.

2.5 Use Traditional Chinese Medicine

During the A (H1N1) pandemic, traditional Chinese medicine and antiserum therapy were also introduced. A prospective randomized and controlled clinical trial was conducted in four provinces in China. The results showed that oseltamivir and maxingshigan-yinqiaosan, alone and in combination, reduced the time to bring down a fever in patients with H1N1 influenza virus infection. These data suggested that maxingshigan-yinqiaosan might be used as an alternative treatment to H1N1 influenza virus infection [11].

2.6 Strengthen Risk Communication and Health Education

China considered active communication with media as one of the most important measures for pandemic response. Public information and risk communication messages were disseminated through a variety of media, including television, radio, and extensively distributed printed materials.

China has set up a regular mechanism to timely release epidemic information and prevention and control progress and established a 24/7 hotline 12320 to reply to inquiries. More importantly, it was very useful to monitor public opinions, make real-time analysis, and adjust media policy in time. These measures played an important role in maintaining public social harmony and stability.

3. Experience and Lessons Learned

3.1 An Influenza Pandemic Can Occur Anywhere in the World and in Any Season

Before the 2009 pandemic occurred, people assumed that Southeast Asia might be the epicenter of influenza pandemics. This hypothesis was supported by the 1957 Asian H2N2 and the 1968 Hong Kong H3N2 pandemics. However, the pandemic H1N1 2009 originating from Mexico indicates that it can emerge anywhere in the world. Therefore, global influenza surveillance and preparedness for influenza pandemics need to continue.

3.2 A Functional and High-Quality Surveillance System Is the Foundation for Epidemic Response

By 2005, the influenza surveillance system, established in China in 2000, had expanded to 63 network laboratories and 197 sentinel hospitals in 31 provinces. In 2009, in order to respond to the pandemic, the system further expanded to more than 400 network laboratories and 556 sentinel hospitals, thus covering all prefectures/cities and priority counties throughout the country. The surveillance system could perform real-time PCR and virus isolation, and the isolated viruses were sent to CNIC for further identification, via genetic sequencing, antigen analysis, etc. to provide timely evidence for risk assessment.

3.3 Joint Emergency Response Mechanism and Hierarchical Prevention Strategy Are the Keys to the Scientific and Efficient Response

A joint prevention and control working mechanism led by the Ministry of Health and joined by 33 departments is the core of overall responses to the H1N1 pandemic 2009, especially in terms of the vaccine development and related trials. This mechanism ensured the establishment of a strong leadership before the pandemic virus spread to China, the development of an integrated approach to coordinate actions taken by different departments, and the management of information sharing and risk communication in a timely and accurate manner. With the progress of the pandemic, China adopted a hierarchical prevention strategy under the "joint prevention and control" mechanism to stringently prevent the imported cases in the early stage and focus on severe cases in the later stage.

Pandemic H1N1 2009 was the first pandemic in the twenty-first century but will definitely not be the last one. One of the most important legacies from the 2009 pandemic response is the expanded national influenza surveillance network, which is critical for quick detection of any pandemic potential influenza virus in China. There is a need to continually refine and improve influenza identification, prevention, and treatment options to prepare for the next pandemic.

Prevention and Control of Human Infection with H7N9 Avian Influenza in China

1. Overview

On March 31, 2013, China reported the first case of human infection with H7N9 avian influenza in the world. After that, the National Health and Family Planning Commission announced that it would include H7N9 in China's notifiable category B infectious diseases for management. As of October 2019, China mainland had reported a total of 1537 cases and 612 deaths of avian influenza A (H7N9), with a fatality rate of 39.8%. The avian influenza H7N9 virus has been clarified as a new gene reassortant virus that could infect humans across species barriers and cause morbidity and death. It was a strong warning for China and global prevention and control of emerging infectious disease and influenza pandemic preparedness. Although the H7N9 avian influenza was only endemic in China and effectively controlled, the H7N9 avian influenza virus and relevant epidemic have attracted widespread attention from domestic and international experts.

1.1 Etiology

The avian influenza A (H7N9) virus is a new gene reassortant virus. Its genome is derived from wild bird and poultry influenza gene fragments. H7N9 virus can bind to α-2,3 and α-2,6 sialic acid receptors. As α-2,3 receptors are mainly distributed in the avian digestive tract and human lower respiratory tract, and α-2,6 receptors are mainly distributed in the human upper respiratory tract, it indicates that the H7N9 virus has the ability to bind avian and mammalian cells and its ability to bind α-2,3 receptors is stronger [12, 13]. From March 2013 to October 2016 (the first four epidemic seasons), the H7N9 virus showed low or no pathogenicity to poultry, but most of the human infection presented severe pneumonia. The highly pathogenic H7N9 virus was first detected in H7N9 cases and poultry in late 2016 [14, 15].

1.2 Clinical Features

Human infection with the H7N9 virus causes acute respiratory infections with high severity and mortality. The H7N9 severe cases generally develop rapidly with severe pneumonia occurring most often within 3–7 days of onset. Most of the body temperature remains above 39 °C and often progresses rapidly to acute respiratory distress syndrome (ARDS). The average interval from onset to ARDS in severe cases is 7 days (1–19 days), from onset to shock, 8 days (3–55 days), and from onset to death, 14 days (8–24 days). Most severe cases require admission to the intensive care unit (ICU).

1.3 Epidemiological Characteristics

The new H7N9 virus that causes the human infection is highly homologous to that detected in the live poultry market at the same time. About 60–70% of patients had a clear history of poultry contact. The most likely site of infection was the live poultry retail and wholesale market, a site that provided an ideal place for virus mixing, amplification, and spread of the virus. Exposure to infected chickens is the primary source of human cases. H7N9 virus could be transmitted to individuals through the respiratory tract or close contact with the secretions or excreta of infected poultry and exposure to an environment contaminated by the H7N9 virus. Few cluster cases have been reported, which indicated that the H7N9 virus cannot easily spread from person to person.

Human beings are generally not susceptible to infections by avian influenza viruses. Although a large number of people visit the live poultry market each day, contact or raise live poultry, or engage in poultry-related work, the number of them infected with H7N9 virus or even get sick is still a minority. Therefore, there might be some host factors (such as differences in innate immunity or susceptibility genes) that lead to differences in susceptibility to the H7N9 virus in different individuals. Patients, especially adults or the elderly, get more severe after being infected with H7N9, possibly due to their exposure opportunities, underlying diseases, and autoimmunity.

1.4 Epidemic Overview

Overall, the incidence of the H7N9 epidemic is obviously high in winter and spring. When winter comes, the H7N9 virus becomes active, hence a gradual increase and the first peak of incidence. With the implementation of prevention and control measures such as closing the live-poultry market and restricting cross-regional transport of live poultry, the epidemic level began to decline. As the Spring Festival approached, residents' consumption of live poultry increased, so did the risk of exposure and infection. This led to the second peak of the epidemic, and with the routine market closure in the Spring Festival holiday, the epidemic fell again rapidly. In the winter and spring of 2016 and 2017, the peak of incidence was significantly higher than the historical level. The subsequent epidemic season appeared to be sporadic, which was the lowest level in history.

2. Strategies and Measures of Prevention and Control

After the outbreak of human H7N9 avian influenza in 2013, facing the serious and complex situation of prevention and control, China promptly put forward the overall prevention and control principles, that was, "to attach great importance, be proactive in response, adopt joint prevention and control mechanism, and insist on scientific prevention and control," and formulated a specific prevention and control strategy. Since then, as the epidemic went on and the understanding of the disease deepened, the strategies were adjusted and improved accordingly.

The prevention and control of the H7N9 epidemic in China could be divided into three stages:

First, early emergency response (March 2013 to August 2014), mainly in Eastern China and Southern China. Most of the people infected were from urban areas. The prevention and control work was aimed at the rapid containment of the epidemic. Key measures included establishing and improving joint prevention and control mechanisms at all levels, conducting surveillance, handling outbreak, strengthening the measure of "concentrating experts and resources for concentrated admission of patients," and "early detection, reporting, diagnosis, and treatment." Additional measures, such as the closure of a large number of live poultry markets or the ban on live poultry trading, were adopted in various places.

Second, intensive response (September 2014 to August 2016), when the epidemic was still mainly concentrated in areas of Eastern and Central China. The previous scientific research on the etiology and epidemiology carried out in the first stage helped deepen the understanding of the disease and accumulate some response experience. Further, combined with the epidemic judgment and risk assessment conducted by disease control departments, the control strategies were shifted to reducing the risk of human exposure and infection. The key was to continuously improve the management measures for live poultry, to shift gradually from emergency response to regular and routine control, and to form a live poultry management model suitable for local control. At the same time, local authorities stepped up their efforts on environment surveillance related to poultry and applied the monitoring results to risk assessment, which played an increasingly important role in prevention and control.

Third, continuous strengthening of the exposure control (September 2016 to present). At this stage, the H7N9 virus has shown highly pathogenic mutations in poultry and the epidemic in poultry increased. The epidemic among humans peaked and spread to more than 20 provinces across the country. The number of cases in rural areas has increased significantly. The epidemic rapidly spread to more areas and infect more people. The low-pathogenic and high-pathogenic avian influenza A (H7N9) virus co-circulated in poultry. Thus, the previous control measures could not meet the needs of prevention and control. The agriculture and health departments have reached an agreement on the importance of controlling the H7N9 epidemic in poultry. While further strengthening the management of live poultry sales and wholesale, more and more places have implemented live poultry transport control measures. In addition, poultry vaccination to block the spread of the virus has been carried out to further reduce the risk of human infection from the source.

3. Experience and Lessons Learned

The prevention and control of human infection with H7N9 avian influenza in China has been so far relatively successful. The experience can be summarized as follows:

- Joint prevention and control mechanism, multiple-department cooperation, and scientific decision-making are the cornerstones of a successful response.
- Improved emergency capabilities facilitate the success in early response.
- Technical support is a powerful guarantee for a successful response.
- The control of the epidemic in poultry and the risk of human exposure to the virus is the core of avian influenza epidemic prevention and control.
- Clinical diagnosis and treatment, especially of severe cases, are critical to reducing the harm and impact of the H7N9 epidemic.

There are still many challenges, including inadequate management and control of live poultry transport, poultry vaccination coverage and sustainability, and strong consumer demand for poultry.

In the future, China will continue to carry out successful control measures mentioned above, such as controlling the epidemic in poultry, promoting the transformation and upgrade of the poultry industry, and managing live poultry transport. Influenza virus detection in medical institutions will be promoted for early diagnosis. The development and application of new antiviral drugs should also be on the agenda for avian influenza control.

References

1. World Health Organization. Influenza laboratory surveillance data. https://www.who.int/tools/flunet.
2. WHO. Cumulative number of confirmed human cases of avian influenza A (H5N1) Reported to WHO. https://www.who.int/influenza/human_animal_interface/2019_09_27_tableH5N1.pdf?ua=1. Accessed Oct 30 2019.
3. CDC. Historical reference of seasonal influenza vaccine doses distributed. https://www.cdc.gov/flu/prevent/vaccine-supply-historical.htm. Accessed Oct 30 2019.
4. CDC. Past seasons estimated influenza disease burden. https://www.cdc.gov/flu/about/burden/past-seasons.html. Accessed Oct 30 2019.
5. CDC. Summary of influenza risk assessment tool (IRAT) Results. https://www.cdc.gov/flu/pandemic-resources/monitoring/irat-virus-summaries.htm. Accessed Oct 30 2019.
6. Qin Y, Zhao M, Tan Y, et al. Centennial history of China's influenza pandemic[J]. Chin J Epidemiol. 2018;39(8):1028–31.
7. WHO. Pandemic (H1N1) 2009—Update 112. https://www.who.int/csr/don/2010_08_06/en/. Accessed Oct 30 2019.
8. Dawood FS, Iuliano AD, Reed C, et al. Estimated global mortality associated with the first 12 months of 2009 pandemic influenza A H1N1 virus circulation: a modelling study[J]. Lancet Infect Dis. 2012;12(9):687–95.
9. Xu C, Bai T, Iuliano AD, et al. The seroprevalence of pandemic influenza H1N1 (2009) virus in China. PLoS One. 2011;6:4.
10. Liang X, et al. Saftty and immunogenicity of 2009 pandemic influenza A H1N1 vaccines in China: a multicentre, double-blind, randomised, placebo-controlled trial. Lancet. 2010;375:56–66.
11. Wang C, et al. Oseltamivir compared with the Chinese traditional therapy Maxingshigan-Yinqiaosan in the treatment of H1N1 influenza: a randomized trial. Ann Inter Med. 2011;155:217–25.
12. Shi Y, et al. Structures and receptor binding of hemagglutinins from human-infecting H7N9 influenza viruses. Science. 2013;342:243–7.
13. Zhou J, et al. Biological features of novel avian influenza A (H7N9) virus. Nature. 2013;499:500–3.
14. Zhang F, et al. Human infections with recently-emerging highly pathogenic H7N9 avian influenza virus in China. J Infect. 2017;75:71–5.
15. Liu D, et al. Characteristics of the emerging chicken-origin highly pathogenic H7N9 viruses: a new threat to public health and poultry industry. J Infect. 2018;76:217–20.

7 The Risk, Prevention, and Control of Arthropod-Borne Infectious Diseases

Wei Wu, Xiaoxia Huang, and Jiandong Li

Arthropod-borne infectious diseases usually refer to a group of infectious diseases transmitted among vertebrates and acquired through the bites of infected arthropods. Arthropod vectors with transmission capacity usually include mosquitoes, midges, lice, fleas, ticks, mites, etc., which become infected when they bite a vertebrate infected with a pathogen [1]. The infected vectors can then spread the pathogen to other vertebrates through bites. In the process of transmission, pathogenic organisms enter into the body of the vector organisms, and the spread of disease is furthered by the proliferation of the pathogen in the vector. Some pathogens can invade the egg cells of vector organisms and be transmitted vertically to the offspring. During the development process, the pathogens can be transmitted across stages—if the infected eggs develop into nymphs, larvae, and adults, they carry pathogens, and when they bite and suck blood, they transmit the pathogens to other vertebrates. Therefore, arthropod vectors could play the role of host to carry a pathogen independently in nature without the help of vertebrates for a certain period.

Historically, arthropod-borne infectious diseases have caused serious harm to human beings. With the significant improvement of the global public health system, some arthropod-borne infectious diseases, such as malaria and Japanese B-Encephalitis, have been effectively controlled in most regions. However, with the effects of global warming, the change of ecosystem and environment, and the rapid development of transportation and logistics, the spread of arthropod vectors is more convenient and the areas affected by arthropod-borne infectious diseases are expanding, some conventional infectious diseases are breaking out again, and new arthropod-borne infectious diseases are emerging [2]. According to statistics, arthropod-borne infectious diseases account for 20% of human infectious diseases and 30–40% of deaths due to infectious diseases.

W. Wu · X. Huang · J. Li (✉)
National Institute for Viral Disease Control and Prevention, China CDC, Beijing, People's Republic of China
e-mail: ldong121@126.com

W. Yang (ed.), *Prevention and Control of Infectious Diseases in BRI Countries*, https://doi.org/10.1007/978-981-33-6958-0_7

Arbovirus is an arthropod-borne pathogen most easy to spread globally, especially in terms of infectious diseases transmitted through *Aedes* mosquitos. There are many kinds of arboviruses. They are widely distributed, but the most closely related to human beings are the viruses in the family of *Flaviviridae*, *Togaviridae*, *Peribunyaviridae, Phenuiviridae*, and *Reoviridae*. When a human being is infected by one of these viruses through mosquitos biting, the clinical manifestations are similar—mainly fever and rash, with or without severe symptoms, such as hemorrhage, shock, and encephalitis. In recent years, areas that are directly affected by these viruses, and in particular, yellow fever virus (YFV), dengue virus (DENV), Zika virus (ZIKV), chikungunya virus (CHIKV), and Rift Valley fever virus (RVFV), are expanding. They are mainly transmitted by *Aedes* mosquitoes, and have attracted worldwide attention.

7.1 The Prevalence of Arthropod-Borne Infectious Diseases in "Belt and Road" Countries

7.1.1 Dengue Fever

Dengue fever is an acute infectious disease caused by the dengue virus, which is spread to people through the bite of an infected *Aedes* species (*Ae. aegypti* or *Ae. albopictus*) mosquito. It spreads rapidly and is one of the most serious arthropod-borne infectious diseases in tropical and subtropical areas. According to the statistics of the World Health Organization, about 2.5 billion people from more than 100 countries and regions around the world live in areas with a risk of dengue [3].

Dengue virus belongs to the flavivirus of the *Flaviviridae* family. Of the four types of viruses, dengue fever can be caused by anyone of them. Different types of dengue virus can circulate in a region simultaneously or sequentially, which increases the incidence of severe dengue fever and its mortality. The natural hosts of the virus are human beings and nonhuman primates, and the main vectors are *Aedes aegypti* and *Aedes albopictus*. In urban areas, the virus circulates between humans and *Aedes* mosquitoes, and in forest areas of Southeast Asia and West Africa, the virus circulates between nonhuman primates and mosquitoes. With the general trend of global warming, dengue fever is showing an increasing trend and the incidence rise rapidly. The number of reported cases increased by more than 30 times in the past 50 years.

In 1779, the outbreak of suspected dengue fever, known as "bone fracture fever" or "bone pain fever," was first reported in Jakarta, Indonesia, and Cairo, Egypt. In 1944, Sabin and others first isolated dengue I and II viruses from soldiers in Indonesia and Hawaii. In 1956, Hammon and other isolated dengue III and IV viruses in the Philippines.

At present, dengue fever is prevalent around the year in Southeast Asia and South Asia. Four serotypes of dengue virus are endemic simultaneously, showing periodicity of 2–5 years. A small number of dengue fever cases and severe dengue like cases have also been reported in the Arabian Peninsula. In Africa, there are also four types of dengue virus endemic, among primates and humans, and dengue fever is prevalent in most of the urban population in West Africa. Since 1977, four serotypes of dengue virus have been introduced into tropical and subtropical areas of the Americas and local transmission has been established. Since 1981, dengue virus have been found in Pacific island countries and Oceania countries, like Australia. By the late 1990s, more serotypes of dengue virus were endemic or cyclical in the Caribbean and Latin America. In 2019, the global dengue fever epidemic shows a trend of high incidence, especially in Southeast Asia, South Asia, and Latin America, and the incidence peaked in many countries in the same period of history.

In China, the prevalence of dengue-like diseases can be traced back to 1873, when more than 75% of people in Xiamen fell ill. At the beginning of the twentieth century, dengue-like outbreaks occurred in Shanghai, Hangzhou, Guangzhou, Hankou, etc. However, the first laboratory-confirmed outbreak occurred in 1978, and outbreaks caused by Type 4 dengue virus were reported in Guangdong Province [4]. In the next 10 years, over 10,000 cases were reported annually in 6 years, among which over 400,000 cases were reported in 1980, mainly in Guangdong, Guangxi, Hainan provinces [5]. By 1985, four serotypes of the dengue virus had appeared in China and caused epidemics. Since the 1990s, the disease has been mostly sporadic or small-scale outbreaks caused by imported cases in Southern China. But in 2014, there was a large-scale dengue outbreak in China, with more than 40,000 cases reported. In 2019, while the world was faced with a significantly high incidence of dengue fever, the number of reported cases in China also increased greatly, the areas with local transmission caused by introduced virus expanded northward, but the total number of cases was lower than that in 2014.

7.1.2 Zika Virus Disease

Zika virus disease is an acute viral infectious disease caused by the Zika virus (ZIKV), which is mainly transmitted by *Aedes* mosquito, and generally occurs in tropical and subtropical areas. *Aedes aegypti* is the main transmission vector of ZIKV. *Aedes albopictus*, *Aedes Africans*, and *Aedes flavipectus* can also transmit the virus. At present, it is endemic in Africa, Asia, America, and Pacific island countries. The clinical manifestations of the disease are usually slight and death is rare. However, some cases may have serious consequences, such as nervous system syndrome, infant microcephaly syndrome, and other birth defects or fetal death. It has attracted extensive attention from the world in 2016.

ZIKV was first isolated from monkey serum in the Zika forest of Victoria River in Uganda in 1947, and also from *Aedes Africans* collected in the same area in 1948 [6]. Then, ZIKV was successively isolated from humans and various mosquito vectors. In the early stage, ZIKV disease was mainly distributed in some countries in Africa and Southeast Asia. In 2007, there was a large-scale outbreak of ZIKV disease in Yap

Island of the Federated Republic of Micronesia. The main manifestations of the cases were sudden systemic macula or papule, arthritis or arthralgia, or nonsuppurative conjunctivitis. From 2013 to 2014, outbreaks of ZIKV disease occurred in French Polynesia, and syndrome of the nervous system increased among patients, with some patients being diagnosed with Guillain Barré syndrome (GBS). In May 2015, a large-scale epidemic of ZIKV disease appeared in Brazil, which spread rapidly to many countries in the Americas, with a trend of global transmission, and local transmission of ZIKV was found in more than 80 countries or regions. In this epidemic, GBS cases were reported more frequently, and damages in the nervous system, eyes, and hearing were found in infant infection cases. Pregnant women infected with ZIKV may cause infant microcephaly and even fetal death.

Phylogenetic analysis of ZIKV genome sequences using bioinformatics technology showed that the virus might have appeared between 1892 and 1943. Around 1940, the virus spread in Africa twice, forming two sub-genotypes of African type [7]. It spread to Malaysia in 1945, forming Asian type, and to Micronesia in 1960 [8].

In Africa, cases or outbreaks have been reported in Nigeria, Sierra Leone, Ivory Coast, Cameroon, and Senegal in West Africa, Gabon, Uganda, and the Central African Republic in Central Africa. Infant microcephaly and neurological complications caused by ZIKV infection have also been found in Africa. In Asia, ZIKV has been isolated in Singapore, Indonesia, Thailand, Bangladesh, Cambodia, Laos, Malaysia, Philippines, Vietnam, etc., and there have been cases acquired through the local transmission. ZIKV has also been isolated in nature, but no human cases of local transmission have been found in China. In 2007, the first outbreak of ZIKV disease occurred in Yap Island [9]. The virus strain originated from Southeast Asia, which may be introduced by humans, host animals during the period of viremia, or mosquito vectors infected with the virus in tourism and trade activities. In the Americas, Chile confirmed the first case of local infection on Easter Island in February 2014. After that, ZIKV epidemic areas expanded and localized. Outbreaks caused by local transmission were reported in 26 countries and regions, and Brazil and Colombia were the most affected countries.

Imported cases of ZIKV disease from abroad have been found in China, Israel, the United States, Canada, Denmark, Finland, Germany, Italy, Portugal, the Netherlands, Spain, Sweden, the United Kingdom, Slovenia, Switzerland, Austria, Australia, etc. Among them, on January 16, 2016, the United States reported the first microcephaly baby born in Hawaii and infected with ZIKV, whose mother traveled to Brazil when she was pregnant in May 2015.

On February 6, 2016, China mainland found the first imported case, a person who worked in Venezuela in January 2016 [10]. Subsequently, imported cases were found in Guangdong, Zhejiang, Beijing, Jiangxi, Henan, and Jiangsu, and they were mainly from Venezuela, Samoa, Suriname, Guatemala, and other American and Pacific island countries. Researchers have isolated ZIKV from mosquito samples collected in the field of Guizhou and Jiangxi provinces, but no case acquired through local mosquito bites has been reported in these areas.

7.1.3 Yellow Fever

Yellow fever, an acute mosquito-borne infectious disease, originated in Africa and then was brought to America through the slave trade [11]. In 1648, the first recorded outbreak occurred in Yucatan Peninsula, Mexico, and a stable epidemic focus of yellow fever transmission was established in Latin America and South America. Outbreaks of yellow fever were reported in North America and Europe (such as New York, Philadelphia, Charleston, New Orleans, Ireland, England, France, Italy, Spain, and Portugal) in the seventeenth and nineteenth centuries [12].

The spread of *Aedes aegypti* has put many cities at risk of re-emerging of yellow fever [13]. In Africa, endemic areas range from 15° N to 10° S, from the Sahara Desert to northern Angola, the Democratic Republic of Congo, and Tanzania. At present, in Africa, yellow fever is mainly prevalent in 34 countries in sub-Saharan Africa, and there is also a risk of yellow fever epidemic in western and northwest provinces of Zambia. Therefore, in Africa, 27 countries are faced with a high risk of yellow fever epidemic and 8 countries with a medium risk of yellow fever epidemic [14]. Thirteen countries are at high risk of yellow fever endemic in South and Central America [14]. Jungle transmission is limited to tropical areas of Africa and Latin America, with hundreds of cases appearing every year. The vast majority of these cases were young men working in forests or transitional areas, or occupational exposure, in Bolivia, Brazil, Colombia, Ecuador, and Peru, suggesting low vaccination coverage [12]. Historically, yellow fever has occurred in many cities in America, but there has been no outbreak of yellow fever in urban areas of North America for more than 50 years. Yellow fever epidemic in Brazil showed a certain periodicity, characterized as an alternative appearance of a sporadic single case acquired through local mosquitos-mediated transmission, and outbreaks among low immune coverage populations in local areas. The epidemic cycle is generally 3–7 years.

In 2006, WHO and UNICEF launched the "Yellow Fever Initiative," which coordinated yellow fever control activities at the global level, called for endemic countries to integrate yellow fever vaccine into children's immunization programs, launched "Yellow Fever Preventive Mass Vaccination Campaigns" (PMVCs) in high-risk areas, and coordinated the management of stockpiled yellow fever vaccines through the international coordination group on vaccine supply (ICG) to respond to global public health Emergency. The number of yellow fever outbreaks in the world decreased steadily, and no yellow fever outbreaks were reported in Africa in 2015. In 2016, due to the large-scale outbreak of urban yellow fever in Angola and Congo, WHO revised the yellow fever prevention and control initiative and the strategic framework, and proposed the global strategy to "Eliminate Yellow Fever Epidemics" (EYE) in 2017–2026. The strategy includes three strategic objectives: to protect populations at risk, prevent international spread, and contain outbreaks rapidly.

In the past 2 years, the yellow fever epidemic in Nigeria showed a rising trend. Since the Nigerian CDC reported a confirmed yellow fever case to WHO on September 15, 2017, outbreaks of yellow fever have been continuously found in a wide geographical area in Kuala state. From 1 January through 10 December 2019, a total of 4189 suspected yellow fever cases were reported from 604 of 774 Local Government Areas (LGAs) across all the 36 states and the Federal Capital Territory in Nigeria [15].

In China, the first imported yellow fever case was confirmed in Beijing on March 12, 2016, which was also the first imported confirmed case in Asia [16]. In the same year, 11 imported cases of yellow fever were found in China, among whom one died. All of them were business or migrant workers in Angola. So far, no local transmission of yellow fever virus has been found in Asia.

7.1.4 Chikungunya Fever

Chikungunya fever (CHIK) is caused by the chikungunya virus (CHIKV), and transmitted by infected *Aedes* species mosquito bites [17]. It is a self-limited infectious disease characterized by fever and joint pain. CHIKV was isolated for the first time in 1952 during the outbreak in Tanzania; and in Asia, CHIKV was first isolated in 1958 in Thailand [18]. Outbreaks of CHIK in Africa, Asia, including the Indian subcontinent, were then detected and reported. There are 37 countries and regions in the world at risk of endemic or potential endemic of CHIK [17]. The natural hosts of CHIKV are human beings and primates. The main vectors are *Aedes aegypti*, *Aedes albopictus*, and *Aedes Africans*, but the efficiency of different mosquito species in transmission varies significantly. *Aedes aegypti* is a domestic mosquito species with the strongest ability to transmit CHIKV. Based on the genetic analysis of the viral genome, CHIKV is classified into three genotypes, namely West Africa, Asia, and East Central South Africa (ECSA). The virus of each genotype is generally endemic in the corresponding geographical region. From 2005 to 2006, the ECSA virus was introduced into Asia, causing large CHIK outbreaks in the Indian Ocean Islands, India, and Southeast Asia.

People are generally susceptible to CHIKV, and the virus infection rate in susceptible people in the endemic area can be as high as 40–85%. The proportion of patients with latent infection in infected people is not clear. In 2006, India reported more than 1.3 million CHIK cases, but the proportion of asymptomatic infection is very low. Although there are few cases of death directly caused by CHIKV, the monthly reported mortality in the population of CHIK epidemic period is significantly higher than that of the nonepidemic period, suggesting that CHIK may increase the mortality of other diseases.

In China, it is reported that suspected CHIKV virus has ever been isolated from patients, vectors, and bats in Yunnan and Hainan provinces, and antibodies have been detected in humans and some mammalian sera. The first confirmed CHIKV was detected from an imported case introduced from Sri Lanka in 2008, which was an Indian Ocean epidemic strain of ECSA genotype [19]. After that, imported CHIK cases were found in many provinces, but no local transmission of CHIKV was detected before 2010 when an outbreak of local transmission was found in Dongguan City, Guangdong Province, with more than 200 cases reported [20].

7.1.5 Rift Valley Fever

Rift Valley fever (RVF) is a viral zoonosis that affects both animals and humans. RVF virus is a member of the Phlebovirus genus [21]. It was first identified in 1931 during an investigation into an epidemic in sheep on a farm in the Rift Valley of Kenya [21]. Although RVFV often causes severe illness in animals, most people with RVF have either no symptoms or mild illness with fever, weakness, back pain, and dizziness. However, a small percentage (8–10%) of people with RVF develop much more severe symptoms, including eye disease, hemorrhage (excessive bleeding), and encephalitis (swelling of the brain). The early clinical manifestations of RVF are nonspecific, influenza-like disease, fever, headache, myalgia, backache, and other symptoms. The mortality of RVF reported in different epidemic areas varies significantly. Since the discovery of the virus, it has been found in more than 30 countries and mainly in Africa, though there was a large-scale outbreak in Saudi Arabia and Yemen. Imported cases have been reported in Sweden, France, Germany, the Netherlands, Canada, and China.

RVFV was isolated from mosquito vectors in Senegal, West Africa, in 1974. A large-scale outbreak occurred in southern Mauritania in 1987, when 284 cases were reported and 28 people died. An epidemic of RVF among animals was detected in the same year in Burkina Faso. In 1977, a large-scale outbreak occurred in Egypt, outside sub-Saharan Africa, with 18,000 reported cases and 598 deaths [22, 23]. Between 2000 and 2001, the first outbreaks were reported outside Africa, in Saudi Arabia and Yemen [24]. Given the limitation of the public health system in Africa, there was a possibility that the epidemic in some countries was not detected in time. By 2018, the following significant outbreaks had been reported:

An outbreak occurred in Egypt in 1977–1978, when 18,000 cases were reported and 598 people died. The actual number of patients may reach 200,000. The outbreak might be caused by the imported virus through the camel trafficking channel from Sudan, where an intermediate stop was set at Aswan Dam; hence, the epidemic in Egypt. Most of the dead cases had bleeding symptoms, a large number of camels died and pregnant ewes aborted [22, 23].

From 1997 to 1998, it broke out in Kenya and spread to Tanzania and Somalia, when 8000 cases were reported and 350–500 people died. The epidemic spread among camels and sheep, resulting in a large number of deaths [25]. The seroepidemiological survey found that the positive rate of the IgM antibody among residents of the Garissa community in Kenya was 8.9%. In 2000, the first outbreak of Rift Valley fever outside Africa was reported in the Arabian Peninsula, when 1087 cases were reported in Yemen and 121 people died, and 883 cases reported in Saudi Arabia and 124 people died [24]. Outbreaks in Sudan, Kenya, Somalia, and Tanzania in 2006–2007 resulted in more than 900 deaths and a large number of livestock deaths [26]. Compared with the information of the human epidemic, there was an insufficient description of epidemics in animals.

In July 2016, an imported case of Rift Valley fever was confirmed in China [27]. Before the onset of the disease, the patient was engaged in outdoor work in Luanda, the capital of Angola. No outbreak or epidemic of RVF was notified before the infection, suggesting that the risk assessment of RVF could not be only based on the epidemic notification, which to some extent affected the effective identification of cross-border cases.

7.2 The Epidemic Risk and the Principle of Prevention and Control of Arthropod-Borne Infectious Diseases

Health authorities should first clarify the background information of corresponding epidemics of arthropod-borne infectious diseases and molecular epidemiological characteristics of related pathogens in local areas, including at least the dominant species composition of arthropod vectors, the infection rate, and the factors affecting the speed of vector-borne transmission. In addition, with the increasing trend of globalization, logistics, and mobility of people, the introduction of nonnative animals and plants increases on a daily basis. The geographical boundaries of the distribution of some arthropod vectors and insects are broken, and long-distance migration can be completed in a very short time. If they can adapt to the local environment, a new breeding area is then established. In the past 50 years, *Aedes albopictus* has been expanding to all continents in the world and adapted to the environment of most regions. In China, *Aedes aegypti* is mainly distributed in southern Taiwan, Hainan, and some coastal areas of Fujian, Guangdong, and Guangxi. It is also found in border areas of Yunnan Province. *Aedes albopictus* is widely distributed, from Liaoning Province in the north to Shaanxi Province in the northwest, Tibet in the southwest, and 34° in the south. The speed of arboviruses transmission by these mosquito vectors varied with regions, and the adapted evolution of viruses or/and vectors often led to unexpected large outbreaks. Cases of viral pathogen introduction, vector adaptation, and local outbreaks have sounded the alarm for the prevention and control of arthropod-borne infectious diseases worldwide.

The principle for the prevention and control of arthropod-borne infectious diseases is generally based on whether there is an autochthonous transmission of pathogens, vectors, and susceptible populations in the area. A graded response is suggested based on the transmission risk, and emphasis should be put in taking decisive measures to control the scale of the epidemic and prevent the escalation of the epidemic in the early stage. If the local epidemic situation has reached a certain level of, rather than above, the response standard, in principle, the response work can be carried out according to the standard of that level. However, for areas where the previous epidemic situation is very serious, the density of mosquito vectors is particularly high, or there are other factors leading to the high risk of the epidemic spreading; the response work can be launched according to the higher level of standards. Institutions at all levels should adjust response measures in time according to the progress of the epidemic and summarize the epidemic situation of each stage. Countries and regions without local epidemics should pay close attention to the progress of international epidemics and carry out a dynamic risk assessment, improve vaccination services, and health education services for travelers to epidemic countries/regions. They should further implement relevant policies and measures for the inspection of vaccination certificates of people to and from endemic areas of arthropod-borne infectious diseases, keep monitoring mosquito density, release early warning timely, ensure mosquito control, prevention and environment protection, and enhance public health education and professional training.

When an outbreak occurs, comprehensive prevention and control measures should be taken in time in the early stage. These measures mainly include case monitoring and management, *Aedes* surveillance and control, risk assessment and situation study, publicity, education, risk communication, as well as policy, material and funding support. Institutions of disease prevention and control should give full play to their role of technical support in the comprehensive prevention and control, guarantee case and *Aedes* surveillance, timely carry out a risk assessment, situation study, and judgment, and provide scientific and reasonable prevention and control recommendations to administrative departments.

To improve case monitoring and management, first of all, it is needed to formulate technology guidelines of case monitoring and laboratory testing, standardize case report, laboratory rapid testing, verification diagnosis, case investigation, search and treatment, and mosquito prevention and isolation, so as to identify the source of infection, determine the epidemic point, find potentially infected persons, and reduce the severity mortality rate, control the source of infection, and slow down the progress of the epidemic.

There are routine and emergency surveillance and control of *Aedes* mosquito. The surveillance results of *Aedes* should be timely shared and regularly reported to superior disease control agencies. Efforts should be made for mosquito control, environmental clean-up, removal of breeding places, and the effect of these efforts should be dynamically evaluated, and a continuous and effective information notification and feedback mechanism be established. These are the core measures to control *Aedes* mosquito activities and cut off the transmission, and key measures for arthropod-borne infectious diseases prevention and control.

Factors, including the epidemic situation, *Aedes* mosquitos, climate, environment, customs, and culture, risk of introduction, etc., should be comprehensively analyzed for dynamic risk assessment, and the affected administrative areas should be scientifically classified into different levels based on risk assessment, which is the core technical support to target the prevention and control measures.

Publicity, education, and risk communication should be carried out in a wide and in-depth way through media, network, communication, teaching, and other ways, so as to give timely early warnings, communicate risks, and popularize disease-related knowledge. Fully mobilize communities, clear the breeding ground of mosquito vectors, and form the habit of mosquito prevention and control, which is a vital part in the prevention and control of mosquito-borne infectious diseases.

According to the response preparedness of the region, governments at all levels should prepare well in personnel, funds, materials, logistics, transportation, and other supports. It is the fundamental requirement for the prevention and control work. The epidemic prevention and control measures should be implemented in accordance with the government leadership and multi-departmental cooperation mechanism. Based on previous experience, the main departments involved include public health, health care, publicity, housing and construction, urban management, education, tourism, public security, finance, inspection and quarantine, etc. The disease control agency can recommend the government to carry out comprehensive prevention and control with reference to the following:

Disease prevention and control institution: carry out epidemic monitoring, *Aedes* mosquito monitoring and assessment, analyze the epidemic situation, carry out epidemic analysis and risk assessment, put forward prevention and control measures and suggestions, and provide technical support for all aspects of the prevention and control work.

Public health administration: be responsible for leading and coordinating medical, public health, health care, health supervision, health education, and other institutions, provide technical support, coordinate experts, strategies, suggestions, etc.

Environmental department: carry out mosquito control, environmental treatment, and elimination of breeding places of *Aedes* mosquitoes, conduct environmental health quality inspection, supervision, and evaluation, and implement the accountability system.

Medical institution: be responsible for the diagnosis, isolation, treatment, and management of cases, sampling, laboratory testing or delivery to qualified laboratories for testing, case report, assistance in case investigation and epidemic analysis, training of medical staff in disease-related knowledge and personal protection, nosocomial infection control, health publicity and education, and case psychological guidance.

Health supervision institution: supervise and inspect the prevention and control of infectious diseases according to relevant laws and regulations.

Health education institution: cooperate with the propaganda department to disseminate diseases prevention and control knowledge, and focus on providing technical support for health communication.

Publicity department: carry out publicity and education on infectious diseases, public opinion tracking and guidance, epidemic reporting, risk communication, and mass mobilization.

Housing and construction department: be responsible for the environmental sanitation management and mosquito control and prevention at construction sites, residential areas, municipal and green facilities, pipeline, and sewage systems, strengthen environmental cleaning and garbage removal, and assist in the management of secondary water supply and mosquito prevention.

Education department: be in charge of mosquito control (killing adult mosquitoes and removing stagnant water) in schools and kindergartens, publicity and education for teachers and students, and call for mosquito control at home.

Urban administration: actively cooperate with environmental, housing, and construction departments to strengthen the supervision and inspection of the environmental health at construction sites.

Tourism department: organize subordinate organizations to publicize knowledge on infectious disease prevention and control, and timely contact relevant departments to handle suspected cases.

Public security department: assist and guarantee all departments to carry out prevention and control work.

Financial department: guarantee funds for the prevention and control work.

Inspection and quarantine department: be responsible for quarantine monitoring and infectious disease screening of entry-exit personnel, and cooperate with the health department on a follow-up investigation of suspected cases found at the port and their close contacts.

Governments at all levels may, according to the actual situation of the region and the needs of epidemic prevention and control, include other departments in the multi-sectoral cooperation mechanism for the prevention and control of arthropod-borne infectious diseases.

7.3 Cases of Prevention and Control

Dengue Prevention and Control in China

1. Overview

In China, the mosquito vectors that can transmit dengue virus are widely distributed, among which *Aedes aegypti* is mainly distributed in Hainan, Leizhou Peninsula, Xishuangbanna, Dehong and Lincang City of Yunnan Province, and *Aedes albopictus*, in Liaoning, Hebei, Shanxi, Shaanxi Province, and South China. The first laboratory-confirmed outbreak occurred in 1978. Outbreaks caused by Type 4 dengue virus were found in Guangdong Province, and more than 20,000 cases were reported that year. In the next 10 years, over 10,000 cases were reported annually in 6 years, among which over 400,000 cases were reported in 1980, mainly in Guangdong, Guangxi, Hainan, and other provinces. By 1985, four serotypes of the dengue virus had appeared in China and caused epidemics. Since the 1990s, the epidemic in Southern China has been mostly sporadic or small-scale outbreaks caused by imported cases, and the epidemic situation has remained relatively stable as a whole. The number of reported cases of dengue epidemic peaked in 2014. In 2019, while the world was faced with a significantly high incidence of dengue fever, the number of reported cases in China also increased greatly, the areas with local transmission caused by introduced virus expanded northward, but the total number of cases was lower than that in 2014. Long-term surveillance and field epidemiological investigations revealed preliminarily that the epidemic of dengue in China still features local transmission acquired by dengue viruses introduced abroad, and a stable transmission cycle of dengue virus thus established.

First, the results of virus serotype and genotype monitoring show that all four types of dengue virus infection cases have been introduced into China and caused local transmission, but the virus of the same highly homologous gene subtype has not caused local transmission cases in the same region for 3 consecutive years, and the epidemic situation caused by the same highly homologous gene subtype virus in the same region for 2 consecutive years was also rare. The second is the age distribution of the patients. In China, the majority of the patients are adults, and the proportion of child patients is low. It is accepted that in endemic areas, the proportion of children cases is high, and the proportion of adult cases is low. Third, the results of China's vector surveillance show that the vector density in the southern region peaks in July, but only sporadic local case reports were reported in China, and the local epidemic begins in August, while the epidemics peak in July in Southeast Asia. Virus genome sequence monitoring indicates high consistency with those of the imported viral pathogens. These monitoring results preliminarily suggest that dengue fever has not formed a stable epidemic focus in China. Although there are outbreaks through local transmission every year, they are mainly caused by the rapid establishment of local transmission after the importation of the virus, but the epidemic characteristics do not exclude the risk of a large-scale epidemic of dengue in China. It is inseparable from the fact that China has not formed a stable epidemic focus, thanks to its prevention of the local epidemic of dengue fever for many years in a row, that the government has attached great importance to the prevention and control of dengue fever, effectively implemented measures of prevention and control, and that the living and working conditions of residents have changed rapidly.

2. Prevention and Control Measures

In recent years, China's national dengue prevention and control work mainly include the following measures. After the outbreak of dengue fever in 1978, the Ministry of Health issued the "Dengue Prevention and Control Plan (Trial)" in 1981, which clarified the responsibilities of departments at all levels in the prevention and control of dengue fever, and determined the prevention and control strategies in the hierarchical management of dengue epidemic areas, dangerous areas, and susceptible areas. Technically, the prevention and control measures focused on strengthening epidemic monitoring, dealing with epidemic spots and disease diagnosis and treatment. The laboratory diagnosis program was standardized, and relevant scientific research, publicity, and education for the masses were emphasized.

In 1988, according to the epidemic situation, the Ministry of Health adjusted the dengue prevention and control plan and focused on epidemic reporting, monitoring, mosquito control, epidemic spots treatment, and the strengthening of border quarantine to prevent virus importation. It stressed that measures should be taken according to local conditions. Local governments could formulate specific implementation measures according to the plan in combination with local conditions. Among them, the hierarchical management strategy of key monitoring area and susceptible monitoring area was determined. Coastal areas with frequent or continuous outbreaks of dengue fever were listed as key monitoring areas, long-term monitoring sites were set up, and regular monitoring work should be carried out on vector, pathogen, and human group serology. Areas with *Aedes albopictus* distribution, no case acquired through local transmission reported, but frequent contact with personnel in key monitoring areas was set as susceptible monitoring areas, and the mobile population and vectors were regularly monitored. A comprehensive response system of dengue epidemic reporting, active monitoring, and emergency control were established.

The Ministry of Health issued "Diagnostic Criteria and Principles of Management of Dengue Fever" (Standard of the Ministry of Health, ws216–2001) in 2001 and revised it in 2008. In 2003 and 2008, the Disease Prevention and Control Bureau of the Ministry of Health edited and published the first and second editions of "Dengue Prevention and Control Manual," which updated and standardized the technical problems in specific disease control and prevention. In 2014, the National Health and Family Planning Commission issued guidelines for diagnosis and treatment of dengue fever, and China CDC improved a series of guidelines for dengue prevention and control technology (including case monitoring, laboratory testing, *Aedes* surveillance, *Aedes* control, etc.). In 2015, the epidemic risk of dengue fever in each province was further clarified and divided into three levels, namely, High-risk Area I, Medium-risk area II, and Low-risk Area III, and the "Technical Guidance for Grading Prevention and Control of Dengue" that adhered to the principle of government leadership, multi-sectoral cooperation, joint and mass prevention and control, public and expert integration, and scientific prevention and control was issued. The main purposes of these technical documents were to control the outbreaks at early stages and small scale. The actual goal of prevention and control was to prevent the spread of the epidemic and reduce severe cases and mortality.

3. Experiences and Lessons

Dengue cannot be eliminated, but with proper measures timely adopted in an outbreak, the scale of the epidemic can be effectively contained. Effective prevention and control measures should include rapid case identification, standardized case management, community participation, and community involvement in mosquito vector control, rapid laboratory testing, etc. The case definition for surveillance can be optimized according to the progress of the epidemic and the characteristics of different epidemic areas. Of course, the coordination and leadership of the government, the coordination and action of multiple departments, and the joint prevention and control should never be forgotten.

Yellow Fever Control and Prevention in Nigeria

1. Overview

Nigeria is located in the southeast of West Africa, with a population of 201 million and more than 250 ethnic groups. It is adjacent to Cameroon in the East, Chad Lake in the northeast, Benin in the west, Niger in the north, and Gulf of Guinea in the Atlantic Ocean in the south. The borderline is about 4035 km long and the coastline is 800 km long. The terrain is high in the north and low in the south. There are many rivers in the territory. It belongs to the tropical monsoon climate, which is divided into the dry season and rainy season. The annual average temperature is 26–27 °C. The geographical, climatic environment, and dense vegetation of the country are suitable for the survival and reproduction of *Aedes*, an important vector of yellow fever, and Nigeria accounted for above 90% of all yellow fever cases in the world during 1989 to 1993 [28].

In recent years, Nigeria's overall medical level and public health system have improved significantly, but infectious diseases are still a major public health problem facing the country, and infectious diseases, such as malaria, tuberculosis, AIDS, polio, yellow fever, and Lassa fever, are still important health threats. On September 15, 2017, according to the International Health Regulations (2005), the centers for disease control (CDCs) of Nigeria officially reported a confirmed case of yellow fever in Kuala Prefecture, and from 1 January through 10 December 2019, a total of 4189 suspected yellow fever cases were reported from all the 36 states and the Federal Capital Territory in Nigeria [15].

2. Prevention and Control Measures

According to the reports from WHO, the outbreak response activities in Nigeria are being coordinated by a multi-agency yellow fever Incident Management System (IMS) (15). Assessments were conducted by rapid response teams of local government jurisdictions and national agencies, and problems of low yellow fever vaccination coverage in Nigeria and incomplete routine immunization documentation were identified. Although routine vaccination against yellow fever was included in Nigeria's Expanded Programme on Immunization (EPI) in 2004, most adults are still vulnerable to infection and the overall population has low immunity.

An Emergency Operations Centre (EOC) was activated for the third time, in response to the upsurge of confirmed yellow fever cases reported in a wide-geographic distribution in Nigeria on September 5, 2019, multiple departments and agencies jointly working at CDCs to coordinate and respond to the yellow fever epidemic. The national rapid response team, including experts from the Nigerian CDCs and the National Primary Health Care Development Agency, has been deployed to Bauchi and other affected States to conduct case discovery, case management, and risk communication, mobilize partner support, and provide emergency yellow fever vaccination in important epidemic areas, like Alkaleri, where 407,708 people were vaccinated. Similar campaigns were planned in local government districts adjacent to the affected states.

Nigeria is currently implementing a 4-year (2018–2021) national Preventive Mass Vaccination Campaign (PMVC) plan for yellow fever prevention with the support of GAVI and partners so that all states in the country can be covered. By 2025, the campaign is expected to have been launched in all Nigerian states to protect high-risk groups from yellow fever. This year's phased prevention campaign will be aimed at Anambra, Ekiti, Kazina, and river states, with special activities in Borno. At the same time, the assessment of the states included in the next phase of the plan was started to cope with the epidemic situation. WHO and partners give support to local authorities in implementing these interventions to control the current outbreaks. The yellow fever vaccine is safe and efficient, which can provide lifelong infection protection. As far as international travels are concerned, the International Health Regulations (2005) is revised, and the validity period of relevant international certificates of yellow fever vaccination and the protection period against infection after yellow fever vaccination are changed from 10 years to whole life. As of July 11, 2016, no WHO contracting state shall require international travelers to be vaccinated or vaccinated against yellow fever as a condition of entry, regardless of whether they hold an existing certificate or a new certificate, and regardless of when the certificate was first issued.

3. Experience and Lessons

Nigeria is a high-priority country in the strategy to eliminate yellow fever. Vaccination is the main intervention to prevent and control yellow fever. It is very important to detect and investigate yellow fever cases through strong monitoring as early as possible, so as to control the risk of spread. Prevention of mosquito bites (e.g., insecticides and long clothing) is an additional measure to reduce the risk of yellow fever transmission. The adoption of targeted mosquito vector control measures in cities also helps block transmission.

References

1. Gubler DJ. Resurgent vector-borne diseases as a global health problem. Emerg Infect Dis. 1998;4(3):442–50.
2. World Health Organization. The world health report. Geneva: World Health Organization; 2002.
3. World Health Organization. Dengue guidelines for diagnosis, treatment, prevention and control. 3rd ed. Geneva: World Health Organization; 2009. http://whqlibdoc.who.int/publications/2009/9789241547871_eng.pdf.
4. Qiu FX, Gubler DJ, Liu JC, Chen QQ. Dengue in China: a clinical review. Bull World Health Organ. 1993;71(3–4):349–59.
5. Fan WF, Yu SR, Cosgriff TM. The reemergence of dengue in China. Rev Infect Dis. 1989;11(Suppl 4):S847–53. https://doi.org/10.1093/clinids/11.supplement_4.s847.

6. Dick GW, Kitchen SF, Haddow AJ. Zika virus. I. Isolations and serological specificity. Trans R Soc Trop Med Hyg. 1952;46(5):509–20.
7. Faye O, Freire CC, Iamarino A, et al. Molecular evolution of Zika virus during its emergence in the 20(th) century. PLoS Negl Trop Dis. 2014;8(1):e2636. https://doi.org/10.1371/journal.pntd.0002636.
8. Haddow AD, Schuh AJ, Yasuda CY, et al. Genetic characterization of Zika virus strains: geographic expansion of the Asian lineage. PLoS Negl Trop Dis. 2012;6(2):e1477. https://doi.org/10.1371/journal.pntd.0001477.
9. Duffy MR, Chen TH, Hancock WT, et al. Zika virus outbreak on Yap Island, Federated States of Micronesia. N Engl J Med. 2009;360(24):2536–43. https://doi.org/10.1056/NEJMoa0805715.
10. Li J, Xiong Y, Wu W, et al. Zika virus in a traveler returning to China from Caracas, Venezuela, February 2016. Emerg Infect Dis. 2016;22(6):1133–6. https://doi.org/10.3201/eid2206.160273.
11. Monath TP. Yellow fever. In: Monath TP, editor. The arboviruses: epidemiology and ecology. Boca Raton, FL: CRC Press; 1989. p. 139–232.
12. Monath TP. Yellow fever: an update. Lancet Infect Dis. 2001;1(1):11–20.
13. Tomori O. Yellow fever: the recurring plague. Crit Rev Clin Lab Sci. 2004;14(4):391–427.
14. WHO. A global strategy to eliminate yellow fever epidemics 2017–2026. Geneva: World Health Organization; 2018. Licence: CC BY-NC-SA3.0 IGO.
15. WHO. Yellow fever—Nigeria. Disease outbreak news: update. https://www.who.int/csr/don/17-december-2019-yellow-fever-nigeria/en/.
16. Chen Z, Liu L, Lv Y, et al. A fatal yellow fever virus infection in China: description and lessons. Emerg Microb Infect. 2016;5(7):e69. https://doi.org/10.1038/emi.2016.89.
17. World Health Organization (WHO). Guidelines for prevention and control of chikungunya fever. [17 August 2013]. http://www.searo.who.int/entity/emerging_diseases/topics/Chikungunya/en/index.html.
18. Robinson MC. An epidemic of virus disease in Southern Province, Tanganyika Territory, in 1952–53. I. Clinical features. Trans R Soc Trop Med Hyg. 1955;49:28–32.
19. Zheng K, Li J, Zhang Q, et al. Genetic analysis of chikungunya viruses imported to mainland China in 2008. Virol J. 2010;7:8. https://doi.org/10.1186/1743-422X-7-8.
20. Wu D, Wu J, Zhang Q, et al. Chikungunya outbreak in Guangdong Province, China, 2010. Emerg Infect Dis. 2012;18(3):493–5. https://doi.org/10.3201/eid1803.110034.
21. Nanyingi MO, Munyua P, Kiama SG, et al. A systematic review of Rift Valley Fever epidemiology 1931–2014. Infect Ecol Epidemiol. 2015;5:28024.
22. Johnson BK, Chanas AC, Tayeb E, et al. Rift valley fever in Egypt, 1978 [J]. Lancet. 1978;312(8092):745. https://doi.org/10.1016/S0140-6736(78)92753-8.
23. Hoogstraal H, Meegan JM, Khalil GM, et al. The Rift Valley fever epizootic in Egypt 1977–1978. 2. Ecological and entomological studies.[J]. Trans R Soc Trop Med Hyg. 1979;73(6):624–9. https://doi.org/10.1016/0035-9203(79)90005-1.
24. Madani TA, Al-Mazrou YY, Al-Jeffri MH, et al. Rift valley fever epidemic in Saudi Arabia: epidemiological, clinical, and laboratory characteristics[J]. Clin Infect Dis. 2003;37(8):1084–92. https://doi.org/10.1086/378747.
25. Woods CW, Karpati AM, Grein T, McCarthy N, et al. An outbreak of Rift Valley fever in Northeastern Kenya, 1997–98. Emerg Infect Dis. 2002;8(2):138–44.
26. Hassan OA, Ahlm C, Sang R, et al. The 2007 rift valley fever outbreak in Sudan[J]. PLoS Neglected Trop Dis. 2011;5(9):e1229.
27. Li M, Wang B, Li L, Wong G, et al. Rift valley fever virus and yellow fever virus in urine: a potential source of infection. Virol Sin. 2019;34(3):342–5. https://doi.org/10.1007/s12250-019-00096-2.
28. Robertson SE, Hull BP, Tomori O, et al. Yellow fever: a decade of reemergence. JAMA. 1996;276(14):1157–62.

8 Plague Risk and Prevention

Xiaona Shen and Wei Li

Plague is a severe infectious disease caused by *Yersinia pestis*. It is primarily a disease of wild rodents and humans get infection mainly by direct contact with the tissues of an infected animal or by bite of an infected flea. Three worldwide plague pandemics had occurred in history, causing hundreds of millions of death [1], which affected the progress of civilizations of human beings. The natural plague foci are widely distributed in many areas of the world [2]. Traced by lineage-specific single nucleotide polymorphisms (SNPs), phylogenetic analysis showed that *Y. pestis* evolved in East Asia, then spread to the rest of the world including Europe, Africa, South America, and Southeast Asia [3]. Most human cases of plague occurred in areas of natural plague foci [4]. At present, the known natural plague foci are distributed in more than 50 countries in Asia, Africa, and the Americas. Even in some countries, such as Madagascar and the Democratic Republic of Congo, plague epidemics are still serious [4]. Cost-effective management and sustainable preventive strategies should be adopted to deal with the re-emerging of plague, which is threatening the modern world [5].

8.1 Overview of the Plague Epidemic in the World

According to the data of the World Health Organization, there were 28 countries in the world that reported a total of 54,352 cases of human plague from 1990 to 2018 [6–8]. These countries, 13 were in Africa (Madagascar, Zambia, Uganda, Botswana, Kenya, Malawi, Zimbabwe, Mozambique, Libya Arab Jamahiriya, Namibia, United

X. Shen · W. Li (✉)
National Institute for Communicable Diseases Control and Prevention, China CDC, Beijing, People's Republic of China
e-mail: liwei@icdc.cn

W. Yang (ed.), *Prevention and Control of Infectious Diseases in BRI Countries*, https://doi.org/10.1007/978-981-33-6958-0_8

Republic of Tanzania, Democratic Republic of Congo, and Algeria), ten in Asia (China, India, Kazakhstan, Mongolia, Viet Nam, Myanmar, Laos, Russian Federation, Kyrgyzstan, and Indonesia), and five in the Americas (Brazil, Bolivia, Peru, Ecuador, and the United States).

Entering into the Twenty-first century, according to WHO statistics, human plague continued showing a high incidence worldwide. From 2000 to 2009, a total of 21,725 human plague cases with 1612 deaths were reported [6]. The countries that recently occurred plague outbreaks included Uganda, China, the Democratic Republic of Congo, the United States, and Madagascar, et al. In terms of geographical distribution of plague, Africa is the most serious epidemic region. From 2000 to 2009, there were a total of 21,064 cases in Africa with 1558 deaths, accounting for 96.96% and 96.65% of the total cases and deaths in the world, respectively [6]. From 2000 to 2009, a total of 234 cases of human plague with nine deaths were reported in the Americas, and 437 human cases of plague with 46 deaths were reported in Asia [6]. More than 90% of the plague cases occurred in Africa in the last two decades, particularly in Madagascar, democratic Congo [6–8]. The most recent plague outbreak occurred at the Uganda–Congo border on March 5, 2019 [9].

From August to November 2017, Madagascar experienced a large pneumonic plague outbreak [10]. The plague outbreak mainly occurred in two large cities, Antananarivo, the capital, and Toamasina, a western port city. A total of 2417 cases with 209 deaths (fatality rate 8.6%) were reported in Madagascar in 2017, including 1854 pneumonic plague patients (76.7% of the total confirmed cases), 355 bubonic plague cases (14.7%), 1 septic plague case, and 207 cases of undetermined infection type [11]. The comparative high fatality rate was attributed to the higher proportion of pneumonic plague in 2017.

Up to 2020, China had identified 12 natural plague foci with different ecological types, which are distributed in 321 counties (cities and banners) in 19 provinces (Autonomous Region). The area of plague natural foci includes about 1.58 million square kilometers [12].

From 2001 to 2020, a total of 252cases of human plague with 44 deaths were reported in China [13], in which four plague outbreaks, whose lessons and experiences are especially worth being remembered. In 2005, An outbreak of pneumonic plague occurred in Yulong County in Yunnan Province. A total of five cases with two deaths were reported. In 2006, the area of the county was identified as a new *Apodemus chevrieri* and *Eothenomys miletus* plague focus [14]. In 2009, an outbreak of pneumonic plague occurred in Qinghai Province. The index patient got infection from an infected dog. A total of 12 cases were involved in the outbreak and three deaths. The event let us profoundly realized the dogs could cause human being's plague infection [15]. In 2014, Three pneumonic plague cases were separately reported in Gansu Province, where belongs to *Marmota himalayana* plague focus in the northern edge of the Qinghai–Tibet plateau [13]. In 2019, there were two pneumonic plague cases and two bubonic plague cases were identified in Inner Mongolia *Meriones unguiculatus* plague focus. In which the two pneumonic plague cases sought treatment in Beijing. The event became the major public health event in China in 2019 for it was the first time that pneumonic plague cases were transported into Beijing since the founding of the People's Republic of China [16]. In next 2020, still in the *M. unguiculatus* plague focus, three human plague cases occurred and two cases died in Inner Mongolia Autonomous Region [13, 17].

8.2 Plague Risk and Prevention and Control Principles

8.2.1 Risk Assessment

Plague is primarily a disease of rodents in corresponding natural plague foci. The disease is transmitted from rodent to rodent via wild rodent fleas, contaminated soil, or cannibalism. Infected fleas play important role in transmission to human plague. Human plague is more frequently occurred by the bite of an infected flea and occasionally by direct contact with the tissues of an infected animal or inhaling infectious aerosol, such as soil contaminated by *Y. pestis* [16]. Person-to-person transmission typically occurs only among pneumonic plague patients. Wild rodent plague exists in many natural foci, and these plague foci are widely distributed in Continents except Oceania in our earth. Today, there are more than 50 countries of Asia, South America, North America, Africa, and Europe existed natural plague foci [18]. It should be said that the risk of human plague would be persisting as long as the animal plague is active in natural plague foci.

According to the route of infection, plague presents three main clinical forms: bubonic, septicemic, and pneumonic plague. Bubonic plague can further spread to the lungs or blood and cause pneumonic plague, or septicemic plague. Pneumonic plague, the most dangerous form of plague, is highly contagious infectious disease and can spread *Y. pestis* from person to person by airborne droplets. Septicemic and pneumonic plague can lead to a 30–100% of mortality ratio if no timely treatment were admitted [18]. The incubation period of bubonic plague infection is 1–7 days, while the incubation period of pneumonic plague is 1–3 days [18]. So a superficial "healthy personal" who coincidently was being in an incubation period could cause a long-distance dissemination through transportation. In addition, goods, such as goods in container, if it starts shipment from a field located in certain natural plague foci, the infected fleas or rodents in a container could be disseminated from one province to another in a country, or from one country to another country by road, rail, river, and sea.

Modern transportation has greatly facilitated the communication of people and the circulation of materials around the world. However, such convenience also increased the risks of disease spreading. Most of the countries along with the "One Belt and One Road" are developing countries, meanwhile, majority of them have natural plague foci. Therefore, national health services in these countries should work together to better identify the risk of human plague and animal plague, establish communication channels to exchange information about the occurrence of human plague cases and rodent surveillance data, as well as issue early warning bilaterally or multilaterally, carry out joint animal plague investigation, and joint control epizootics in border areas when necessary.

8.2.2 Principles of Prevention and Control

As mentioned above, plague is primarily a disease of wild rodents, while human plague, especially the pneumonic plague, possesses characteristics with high infectivity and fatality. So, comprehensive prevention and control measures should be emphasized. These measures include human plague and animal plague surveillance, epidemiological survey, laboratory timely inspection, and public health education. These measures for prevention and control of plague should be stressed as follows:

1. Prompt reporting. Prompt reporting is especially necessary for human plague cases, especially for the pneumonic plague, because this form of the disease can transmit directly from person to person via infectious aerosols. In China, an information management and report network system for plague surveillance has been established.
2. Strengthen surveillance. Here mentioned surveillance includes human plague monitoring and reservoir surveillance in natural plague foci. Effective human plague monitoring programs include collecting and reporting plague corresponding clinical information from hospitals or clinics, analyses and interprets epidemiological data of plague. On the other hand, continuous and thorough reservoir plague surveillance should be organized within the territory having endemic plague foci. Where all carcasses of rodents should be collected and perform laboratory tests. Such animal plague surveillance aims at detecting plague activity in susceptible rodent populations, assessing potential risk to humans, and issuing an early warning.
3. Patients' quarantine and ensure proper treatment. Patient should be placed in an isolation ward for treatment. It is stressed that patients could obtain appropriate and combined antibiotics treatment, necessary antibiotics susceptibility monitoring of *Y. pestis* should also be performed, especially when treatment failure is suspected due to antibiotic resistance. The corpse of a plague victim should be buried in a safe way. Healthcare staff should be trained and take adequate protective measures when they contact patients or collect samples. According to different situations, the quarantine of close contacts or a *cordon sanitaire* establishing around the infected locality and the field hospital could be considered as soon as the first case of pneumonic plague is detected.
4. Epidemiological investigation. The purpose of this investigation is to obtain detailed exposure history from the patient and further make an initial assessment of likely sources of infection and potential risks to others in certain areas.
5. Control of plague transmission. The most important and effective measure to break the chain of plague transmission is by proper application of effective insecticides. It must be emphasized that immediate control of flea vectors should precede to any measures against rodent hosts, or simultaneously. Because killing rodent hosts may result in the release of large numbers of fleas carrying plague organisms seek new hosts. Such a campaign actually is an eco-

logical disturbance activity, and it increases corresponding risk that free fleas inhabited in focus to attack humans. In addition, insecticide susceptibility tests must be done to determine the status of resistance of the flea populations and for selecting insecticides used. Once flea indices have been reduced, control of rodent reservoirs can be undertaken. In fact, the control of rodents in rural areas is a more difficult undertaking. The way of using proper rodenticides is only one of selection for reducing the rodent population. The most effective methods of reducing the rodent population in human dwelling are comprehensive public health campaign, including improvement in sanitation, waste disposal, storage of grain, and foodstuffs. It must be emphasized that in order to guarantee the efficiency of controlling plague rodent reservoirs, it is necessary to evaluate the effect of rodenticides including actual endemic extinguishing effectiveness in an active plague foci.

6. Enhance the ability of laboratory diagnosis. This kind of ability is directed at guaranteeing the surveillance programs are fulfilled smoothly. The process includes timely reservoir specimens shipment, bacteriological examinations, appropriate molecular and serological detection, as well as necessary quality control.
7. Emergency management and response. The successful control and disposal of plague outbreaks, especially for a large-scale epidemic, depends on efficient emergency management and response. This kind of ability should permeate into every corresponding organization at the national, provincial, municipal, and county levels.
8. Public Health Education. Public health education is an important part of plague prevention and control measures. The focus of education should emphasize on "Three Avoid": Avoid hunting and handling rodents, Avoid skinning and eating sick or dead animals, Avoiding take the reservoirs out the endemic locus; "Three Report": Reporting dead reservoirs or its reductions, Reporting suspect plague case, Reporting patient with high fever or die-offs; "Three Preventing": Preventing fleas bites, Preventing cats and dogs getting infected, Preventing ecological disturbance; "Three Applying": Applying insect repellent, Applying insecticides to kill fleas, Applying prophylactic antibiotics [19].
9. Risk assessment and early warning. Up to now, there is no fully risk communication among countries threatened by plague, including lack of risk communication after occurrence of human plague cases and lack communication on animal plague surveillance. It is necessary to lay emphasis upon risk assessment based on animal plague surveillance. In addition, early warning should not stay only on documents, but should tell the public and corresponding health authorities. Such measures could allow prevention and control programs to be implemented before human plague cases occurred.
10. Scientific research and technology communication. There should be a consensus that bilateral or multilateral scientific cooperation and technical communication could promote the world professionals unite and co-deal with plague epidemics or international transmission, which will great benefits the plague surveillance, risk assessment, early warning, and outbreak control.

8.3 Plague Control Cases

Case 1: Treatment of Plague in Yunnan, China, in 2016

1. **Overview**

In 2016, a human case of plague was reported in Yunnan Province [20]. The patient (female, 68 years old) was a retired worker from a farm in Puwen Town, Jinghong City. The initial symptoms of the patient included fever, fatigue, poor appetite, and malaise for several days. Thereafter, on June 1, she was admitted to the local hospital with a high fever (39.5 °C), accompanied by chills, sweating, nausea, vomiting, and coughing occasionally. No expectoration and hemoptysis were complained by the patient, and her pulse rate was 87 times/min, breath rate was 19 times/min, blood pressure was 130/50 mmHg; in addition, no swelling of superficial lymph node was detected and there was no obvious rale in the lungs; the X-ray chest film presented a common image of chronic bronchitis; WBC was 13.13×10^9/L, the absolute value of neutrophils was 12.2×10^9/L, the percentage of neutrophils was 92.91%; The bacterial culture of throat swab was reported as *Candida albicans*; but the vein blood culture was reported as *Yersinia pestis*. The patient recalled that she once collected dead commensal rats (local reservoirs, *R. flavipectus*) from a chicken house without any protection about 15 days ago [21]. The patient was finally diagnosed with primary septicemic plague and she was cured on June 18, 2016 [20].

According to the epidemiological investigation, a total of 58 close contacts of the patient, including four medical staff in the village clinic, 16 relatives or immediate family members, 11 neighbors, and 27 medical staff in Jinghong People's Hospital [21], were put in quarantine and medical observation. No abnormality was found in these contacts. According to reports from the residents in same community, the phenomenon of dead rats had appeared in the community since mid-May. During June 11–13, the field survey team in local CDC collected four dead rats (*Rattus flavipectus*) in the community. The reverse indirect hemagglutination tests for these rat's organs specimens were positive, and two *Y. pestis* strains were isolated from these carcass specimens. So the area outbreak that occurred was determined as a re-active *R. flavipectus* plague focus, for there once occurred human plague epidemics in Jinghong County in Yunnan Province in the 1980s and 2008 [21].

2. **Prevention and Control Measures**

The local government and relevant departments performed a comprehensive prevention and control measures to cope with the public health event, as follows:

First, the local government strengthened the organizational leadership. Corresponding plans associated with prevention and control were formulated. The local government established an epidemic prevention and control headquarters with the government leaders as commander, and ten professional and technical groups were organized, such as epidemiological investigation, inspection, public health campaign, rodenticide and insecticide, information notification, laboratory testing, and media publicity group. On one hand, the headquarter assigned concrete assignments to corresponding groups, on the other hand, the headquarters guided and inspected implementation of these measures.

Second, laboratory testing and patient treatment were strengthened. National, provincial, and municipal microbiological laboratories joined together to guarantee specimens from animals or patients were tested timely. A professional medical treatment team in the local hospital was organized for patient treatment.

Third, professional personnel were deployed to carry out epidemiological surveys. All close contacts were identified through such investigation. In this event, a total of 58 close contacts were quickly identified, and a 9-day home quarantine and medical observation were conducted. In order to strengthen the ability of information notification, an active fever patient searching campaign was performed, and a zero-reporting system of patients with fever with unknown causes was also initiated.

Fourth, a comprehensive public health campaign including rodenticide and insecticide measures were implemented to control plague epizootics. In order to guarantee the best effectiveness for breaking the chain of plague transmission, four concrete steps of public health measures were performed, as follows: performing public health and environmental cleaning campaign; conducting effective insecticides; killing rodent hosts by rodenticides; and application insecticides again. Next, the assessment of endemic extinguishing effectiveness was carried out to inspect the effect of above prevention and control measures.

In addition, an enhanced rodents surveillance, as well as health promotion and education was also carried out to consolidate these measures.

3. **Prevention and Control Experience**

The situation that the human plague epidemics had been successfully controlled in China benefitted from the efficient emergency management in China. In which, the first and most important experience in successful control of plague outbreaks lies in dealing with the plague epidemics according to corresponding infectious disease prevention and control laws and technical standards. Corresponding national regulations associated with public health emergency disposal provided a legal basis for plague emergency management when plague epidemic occurred. In such a situation, the local government burdens the responsibility to prevent and control plague outbreaks. In addition, local government coordinates all related departments, such as traffic units, public security agents, CDC, and hospital to respond quickly and more effectively. Through above-mentioned plague emergency management system, governments at all levels could ensure corresponding comprehensive prevention and control measures be carried out efficiently.

Case 2: Plague Epidemic in Madagascar in 2017

1. **Overview**

In 2017, Madagascar suffered an urban pneumonic plague epidemic in the capital city Antananarivo and major western city Toamasina [10]. From August 1 to November 26, a total of 2414 cases, contained confirmed, probable, and suspected cases of plague, were reported in Madagascar, including 202 deaths, with a case fatality rate of 8.6% [10]. The weekly number of reported pneumonic plague cases increased significantly at the end of September 2017, reaching a peak of 423 cases in the week beginning on October 2, 2017. On November 27, 2017, the Health

Ministry of Madagascar announced the urban pneumonic plague outbreak was controlled.

Among these plague cases, there were 1878 cases of pneumonic plague, 395 cases of bubonic plague, 140 cases of no clinical types plague, and 1 septicemic case. Of the 1878 pneumonic plague cases, 32 were confirmed (2%) and 386 (21%) were probable plague cases. Of the 395 bubonic plague cases, 66 were confirmed cases (17%) and 73 (18%) were probable cases [10]. Only about 50 strains of *Y. pestis* were isolated totally. All strains were sensitive to the antibiotics following Clinical Laboratory Standards guidelines. Pneumonic plague occurs mainly in the cities of Antananarivo (288 / 418, 69%) and Toamasina (63 /418, 15%), with significant spatial clustering. The bubonic plague cases increased and peaked in the same period as pneumonic plague [10]. Of the 139 confirmed or probable cases of bubonic plague, 131 (94%) occurred in plague endemic areas that contained 31 districts in Antananarivo [10].

2. **Prevention and Control Measures**

The Madagascar's Public Health Ministry cooperated in response, with the aid of WHO, the Pasteur Institute of Madagascar, and other international agencies (China also organized and dispatched two expert teams to Madagascar). The Madagascar's Public Health Ministry launched emergency response field teams in Antananarivo and Toamasina to deal with the outbreak. The public health response measures are as follows [10, 11]:

1. All patients were placed in the isolation wards for treatment with sufficient doses of antibiotics, and all patients and contacts received treatment or prophylactic antibiotics.
2. Quick investigation of new cases was undertaken, strengthened epidemiological surveillance in all epidemic areas, including strengthening case detection, actively sought, tracked, monitored contacts, and provided free prophylactic antibiotics.
3. Vector and animal control was performed, including proper pesticides and public sanitation.
4. Collected, transferred, and tested samples. Applying rapid detection technology to improve diagnostic accuracy.
5. Improved public awareness of the prevention of plague; provided suggestions about infection control about funeral; improved awareness of medical staff and provide suggestions to promote case detection and protective measures.
6. Import and export port screening measures were implemented at Antananarivo and Nocibe International airports to prevent the international spread of pneumonic plague cases.

3. **Prevention and Control Experience**

The Madagascar plague in 2017 was a typical urban pneumonic plague epidemic. The epidemic had a huge impact on the economy and society in Madagascar in 2017. The plague epidemic in Madagascar came earlier in 2017. In previous years, the plague usually happened from October to April of next year, but in 2017, it began in August. Patients were mostly concentrated in large central cities, with plague outbreaks occurred in some epidemic and non-epidemic regions. The intensity of the bubonic plague cases was basically the same as in previous years, but the intensity of pneumonic plague cases far exceeded that in previous plague epidemics in Madagascar. Because urban pneumonic plague and human-to-human transmission presented multipoint outbreaks in Madagascar and the pneumonic plague has a high fatality rate, so rapid and comprehensive measures were the key for controlling the urban pneumonic plague epidemic in Madagascar in 2017.

In this plague epidemics, WHO was invited to support corresponding breakout control. WHO sent more than 100 experts for assistance. Many countries or organizations also participated in the epidemic treatment. According to the published literature [10], lack of laboratory testing capabilities in the field should be the reason that too many untyped cases were reported in this epidemic. In addition, there lacks continually and systematic reservoirs plague surveillance in Madagascar.

References

1. Perry RD, Fetherston JD. *Yersinia pestis*-etiologic agent of plague. Clin Microbiol Rev. 1997;10:35–66.
2. Zietz BP, Dunkelberg H. The history of the plague and the research on the causative agent *Yersinia pestis*. Int J Hyg Environ Health. 2004;207:165–78.
3. Morelli G, Song Y, Mazzoni CJ, et al. Phylogenetic diversity and historical patterns of pandemic spread of *Yersinia pestis*. Nat Genet. 2010;42:1140–3.
4. Yang R, Anisimov A. *Yersinia pestis*: retrospective and perspective. Dordrecht: Springer; 2016.
5. Ditchburn J-L, Hodgkins R. *Yersinia pestis*, a problem of the past and a re-emerging threat. Biosaf Health. 2019;1:65–70. https://doi.org/10.1016/j.bsheal.2019.09.001.
6. Weekly Epidemiological Record (WER), No. 6. 2010;85:37–48.
7. Weekly Epidemiological Record (WER), No. 8. 2016;91:89–104.
8. Weekly Epidemiological Record (WER), No. 25. 2019;94:289–292.
9. Aljazeera. WHO: deadly plague breaks out on Uganda-Congo border. 2019. https://www.aljazeera.com/news/2019/03/deadly-plague-breaks-uganda-congo-border-190314075949596.html. Accessed 25 Dec 2019.
10. Randremanana R, Andrianaivoarimanana V, Nikolay B, et al. Epidemiologic characteristics of urban plague epidemic in Madagascar, August–November 2017: an outbreak report. Lancet Infect Dis. 2019;19:P537–45. https://doi.org/10.1016/S1473-3099(18)30730-8.
11. https://www.afro.who.int/health-topics/plague/plague-outbreak-situation-reports
12. Zhang G, Tian W, Ju C, et al. Summary of plague surveillance in China in 2019. Chin J Cont Endemic Dis. 2020;35:1–9. (in Chinese)
13. Chinese Information Management System for Plague Control (Internal website). [in Chinese].
14. Wang P, Shi L, Zhang F, et al. Ten years of surveillance of the Yulong plague focus in China and the molecular typing and source tracing of the isolates. PLoS Negl Trop Dis. 2018 Mar 30;12(3):e0006352.
15. Wang H, Cui Y, Wang Z, et al. A dog-associated primary pneumonic plague in Qinghai Province, China. Clin Infect Dis. 2011;52(2):185–90. https://doi.org/10.1093/cid/ciq107. [Epub 2011/02/04, PubMed PMID: 21288842]
16. Wang Y, Zhou L, Fan M, et al. Isolated cases of plague - Inner Mongolia - Beijing, 2019. China CDC Weekly. 2019;1(1):13–6. https://doi.org/10.46234/ccdcw2019.005.

17. Shen X, Li J, Fan M, et al. A Remergent case of bubonic plague-Inner Mongolia Autonomous Region, China, July, 2020. China CDC Weekly. 2020;2(29):549–50. https://doi.org/10.46234/ccdcw2020.145.
18. https://www.who.int/health-topics/plague
19. Li W. Update the plague prevention and control strategy to "three nos, three reports, three cares, three uses". Chin J Epidemiol. 2020;41(3):442–5. [in Chinese]
20. Shi L, Yang G, Zhang Z, et al. Reemergence of human plague in Yunnan, China in 2016. PLoS One. 2018 Jun 13;13(6):e0198067.
21. Shi L, Yang G, Zhao C, et al. Determination and disposal of human plague in Jinghong, Yunnan Province in 2016. Chin J Health Lab Technol. 2017;27(5):1502–7. [in Chinese]

Malaria Risk and Control 9

Sheng Zhou and Zhongjie Li

Malaria is a vector-borne infectious disease caused by infection with plasmodium. It is a life-threatening infectious disease in many tropical and subtropical countries. There are four types of malaria parasites: *Plasmodium vivax, Plasmodium falciparum, Plasmodium malariae*, and *Plasmodium ovale*. *Plasmodium falciparum* is the most harmful to human, followed by *Plasmodium vivax*. It has been found that human beings can be infected by *Plasmodium knowlesi*, which causes malaria in monkeys. Malaria is one of the Class B infectious diseases listed in the "Infectious Diseases Control Law of the People's Republic of China."

9.1 Epidemic Situation in "Belt and Road" Countries

According to WHO statistics, there were 219 million malaria cases in the world in 2017 [1]. It was 217 million in 2016 and 239 million in 2010. Most malaria cases (200 million, or 92%) were reported in the WHO Africa region, 5% in the WHO Southeast Asia region, and 2% in the WHO Eastern Mediterranean Region. The malaria burden of 15 sub-Saharan African countries and India accounted for nearly 80% of the global total. Almost half of the malaria cases in the world were reported from five countries: Nigeria (25%), the Democratic Republic of Congo (11%), Mozambique (5%), India (4%), and Uganda (4%). From 2010 to 2017, the incidence rate of malaria worldwide dropped by 18%, from 72 cases per 1000 people to 59 per 1000 people, and in Southeast Asia, it was 59%, from 17 cases per 1000 people in 2010 to 7 per 1000 people in 2017. *Plasmodium falciparum* is the predominant malaria parasite in the WHO African Region, responsible for 99.7% of the

S. Zhou · Z. Li (✉)
Chinese Center for Disease Control and Prevention, Beijing, People's Republic of China
e-mail: lizj@chinacdc.cn

W. Yang (ed.), *Prevention and Control of Infectious Diseases in BRI Countries*,
https://doi.org/10.1007/978-981-33-6958-0_9

total estimated malaria cases in 2017. It is estimated that 435,000 people died of malaria in 2017. By comparison, the number of malaria deaths was 607,000 in 2010 and 451,000 in 2016. The deaths due to malaria in the WHO Africa region accounted for 93% of all malaria deaths in 2017. Globally, elimination networks are expanding and more and more countries are moving toward zero cases of indigenous malaria. A total of 46 countries reported less than 10,000 cases of malaria in 2017, up from 37 countries in 2010 and 44 countries in 2016. The number of countries with less than 100 cases of indigenous malaria increased from 15 in 2010 to 24 in 2016 and 26 in 2017 [1].

Global malaria response faces many challenges. The immediate obstacle to achieving the 2020 and 2025 milestones of the global malaria technology strategy is the continued increase of malaria cases in countries with the highest disease burden and inadequate international and domestic funding. At the same time, parasite resistance to antimalarial drugs and the continued emergence of mosquito resistance to insecticides also pose a threat to progress.

Malaria prevalence varies widely in "Belt and Road" countries. Despite the continuous decline in reported cases in Ethiopia in recent years, the epidemic is still severe in countries with high malaria burden. According to WHO, Ethiopia reported 7,701,107 malaria cases and 14,514 deaths in 2010 and 2,666,954 malaria cases and 5369 deaths in 2017. The malaria epidemic in Kenya is serious. From 2010 to 2017, 2,845,913; 2,930,265; 3,252,855; 3,754,660; 3,916,556; 3,455,175; 345,217; and 3,520,384 malaria cases were reported respectively, with 11,375; 11,834; 11,990; 12,111; 12,242; 12,331; 12,419; and 12,467 deaths reported respectively. There are countries with no risk of malaria, such as Israel (eliminated), the United Arab Emirates (eliminated), Sri Lanka (eliminated), Kazakhstan, Turkmenistan, etc. Although Malaria burden still exists in many countries in Asia and Oceania, the goal of eliminating malaria by 2030 has been set along with the decline of incidence of malaria in recent years. Malaria is still prevalent in Afghanistan, Pakistan, and India in South Asia.

Malaria was recorded as early as 3000 years ago in China. Before the establishment of the People's Republic of China, malaria was widespread and seriously threatened people's life in China. When new China was first founded, malaria was prevalent in its 1829 (70–80% of the total then) counties. The number of malaria cases was the highest among all kinds of reported infectious diseases [2]. After years of large-scale control, the incidence rate of malaria in China has dropped dramatically. The geographical distribution of four species of Plasmodium has also changed greatly. *Plasmodium ovale* has not been found. Since 1970, only cases of *Plasmodium falciparum* and *Plasmodium vivax* have been reported. Since 1995, indigenous cases of *Plasmodium falciparum* have only been reported in some areas of Yunnan Province and Hainan Province. From 2011 to 2017, 22,305 malaria cases were reported in China, including 105 deaths and 1334 indigenous cases. Most of malaria cases were falciparum malaria (13,377 cases) and vivax malaria (6850 cases) (90.7%). It was the first time that zero indigenous malaria case was reported in 2017 in China, with only 7 cases of deaths reported. The importation from 75 origin countries showed an increasing annual trend from Africa but a decreasing trend from Southeast Asia from 2011 to 2017 [5–12].

9.2 Malaria Risk and Control Principles

9.2.1 Malaria Risk

Despite the progress of global malaria control, the achievements are still fragile and unevenly distributed. Malaria is still prevalent in all six WHO regions. The malaria burden in the African region is the heaviest, accounting for an estimated 90% of global malaria deaths. Millions of malaria patients around the world are still unable to benefit from malaria prevention and treatment, and most cases and deaths from malaria are not registered or reported. Considering the growth of the world population size by 2030, it is expected that more people will live in countries at risk of malaria. Moreover, it is important to keep vigilance and ensure timely detection of disease transmission areas and rapid control, experience learned from malaria-free countries and those having made significant progress in reducing malaria incidence rate and mortality in the past 10 years [3].

9.2.2 Prevention and Control Principles and Measures

WHO proposed three core principles and two supporting elements in the global malaria technology strategy 2016–2030 [3].

The core principles are to:

- Ensure universal access to malaria prevention, diagnosis, and treatment.

  The core interventions package, including quality-assured vector control, chemoprevention, and diagnostic testing and treatment, can dramatically reduce morbidity and mortality. Universal access of populations at risk to interventions should be given top priority in national malaria programs. According to the stratification of malaria, prevention strategies should be based on vector control and universal diagnosis, and prompt and effective treatment of malaria should be available at health facilities of community level.
- Accelerate efforts toward the elimination of malaria.

  Reduce further transmission of new infections in defined geographical areas. In addition to core interventions, active case detection and investigation within foci should be part of malaria surveillance and response.
- Transform malaria surveillance into a core intervention.

  Strengthening malaria surveillance is crucial for accelerating progress. Effective health management and information system should be established. Surveillance should trigger locally tailored response to every detected infection at very low levels of malaria transmission.

The supporting elements are:

- Harnessing innovation and expanding research.

  Successful innovation in product development and service delivery will make a major contribution to accelerating progress. Implementation research will be fundamental to optimize impact and cost-effectiveness and facilitate rapid uptake in populations at risk.

- Strengthening the enabling environment.

  Strong political commitment, robust financing, and increased multisectoral collaboration are key factors for further progress. To optimize national malaria responses, an overall strengthening of health systems and improvement in the enabling environment is also crucial.

  Malaria case-based surveillance was established to strengthen malaria surveillance after the implementation of malaria elimination in China. The strategy of malaria elimination in China was updated as follows in 2019 [4].

- Continue to implement the strategy of "tracking, counting, and cutting off sources" and the work specification of "1-3-7" focusing on eliminating infectious sources and blocking transmission.
- In Yunnan and other border areas with a high risk of malaria transmission, strengthening grass-roots malaria monitoring capacity, multi-sectoral cooperation, cross-border joint prevention and control, and block cross-border transmission of malaria.
- Further strengthening the capacity of malaria monitoring, early warning, and disposal at all levels, enhancing malaria monitoring at the post-elimination and elimination stages, focusing on preventing the risk of retransmission caused by imported malaria, and consolidating the achievements of malaria elimination.

9.3 Case Study

Control Experience of Malaria Importation in Shanglin County

1. Summary

In 2013, a large number of malaria cases were reported in Shanglin County, Guangxi Zhuang Autonomous Region due to the expulsion of Chinese golden miners by the Ghana government. In the face of the risk of malaria transmission brought by large-scale overseas returnees, Shanglin County launched active and effective malaria control and quick response [13, 14]. Details are as follows.

Since June 2013, the number of imported malaria cases has increased significantly in Guangxi Zhuang Autonomous Region, and in particular, in Shanglin County (Fig. 9.1). Cases reported in Shanglin County were on the rise. From May 1 to August 31, 998 malaria cases were reported in Guangxi, among whom 868, or 87.0%, were reported in Shanglin County. All of them were imported malaria cases, and most were falciparum malaria. As of August 31, all the malaria cases reported in Shanglin County had been imported from Ghana, Africa, except one from Indonesia. Of the 868 reported cases, 825 were falciparum malaria (95.0%), 36 were vivax malaria (4.1%), 2 were ovale malaria (0.2%), 1 was malariae malaria (0.1%), 3 were mixed infection (0.3%), and 1 was not classified (0.1%).

Under the coordination and linkage of departments at all levels of the nation, provinces, cities, counties, townships, and villages, the epidemic response was made timely. Under the unified command and with the support of prevention and control personnel, prevention and control materials, and other favorable conditions, efforts were continuously made to screen overseas returnees, fully complete the treatment work, and effectively implement other prevention and control measures, so as to ensure there were no death cases or second-generation cases in this epidemic, and success in the fight against the outbreak.

2. Prevention and Control Practices

1. Establish a leading group for malaria control and organize experts to guide and strengthen the leadership. The County's Party Committee and government attached great attention to the establishment of a malaria prevention and control leading group for overall leadership and coordination of the prevention and control work, and to a daily report by each township during the malaria epidemic period. The provincial health department and CDC of the Autonomous Region assigned officers, malaria control experts, and clinician experts for direct handling of the epidemic on the spot and for technical guidance on prevention and control.
2. Set up malaria screening points for timely detection. The County's Party Committee and government mobilized forces from all townships (towns) and villages to carry out a wide range of screening work for overseas workers returning home and strived to achieve 100% malaria screening rate for these people.
3. Establish treatment points for imported malaria and standardize the treatment of cases. Set up a designated treatment unit, and in particular, increase the number of beds and provide a green channel for malaria reception in the outpatient department for the timely in-hospital treatment of malaria patients. Every malaria patient received standard treatment according to the condition.
4. Manage each focus and conduct active case investigation for residents within the foci.
5. Strengthen the monitoring work. Under the guidance of national and provincial experts, continuous mosquito surveillance was carried out. Blood tests and screening of patients with fever were performed in targeted local residents. Meanwhile, promote and mobilize them to screen Plasmodium at local CDCs or hospitals.
6. Carry out extensive publicity activities. Various forms of mass health education were provided.

3. Experience

There are many inspirations and references from the management of the epidemic for the treatment of similar imported malaria in the future.

1. Governments at all levels attach great importance to the epidemic, and extensive cooperation within multiple departments and sections is the key. Malaria prevention and control work needs overall organization and mobilization of departments at all levels and requires thorough involvement. Communication and cooperation are required within the Inspection and Quarantine Bureau, Public Security Bureau, and other departments. The investigation of migrant workers and returnees in each village can provide relevant data and information, thus ensuring the orderly and effective handling of the epidemic.
2. The reserve of professional and technical capacity in Guangxi provided the scientific and effective technical guarantee for the response to the epidemic. From 2010 to 2012, more than 4000 malaria prevention professionals and technicians were trained, which improved the sensitivity of medical personnel and related malaria prevention personnel, and ensured timely detection and appropriate treatment of malaria cases. It has reserved sufficient technical capacity for the whole region to deal with the malaria epidemic.
3. Centralized testing, designated hospital treatment, and reference laboratories have ensured high-quality control. In order to ensure the quality of the first-line microscopic examination, the blood examination is required to be carried out at the CDC lab or those above the county level for large-scale epidemics. The technical backbone group of the whole region was transferred to Shanglin County for blood examination, so as to minimize potential infectious sources caused by the false negative.
4. By making full use of various means and methods, for instance, with the support of Women's Federation, Shanglin County improved the awareness of returnees and people in the epidemic area of the harm of malaria and enhanced their compliance in the inspection of Plasmodium. It tried to achieve twice the results with half the effort in the prevention and control of the epidemic.

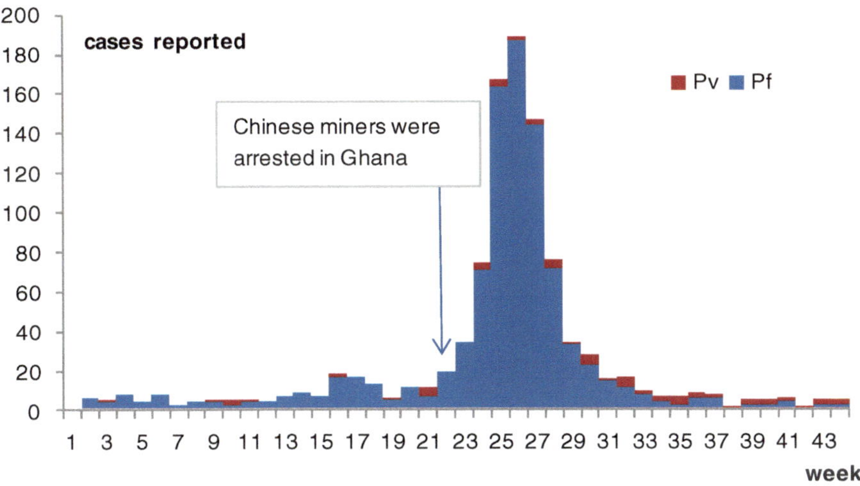

Fig. 9.1 Distribution of reported cases of malaria in Shanglin County, Guangxi, from January to November 2013

References

1. WHO. 2018. World Malaria Report 2018.
2. Tang LH, Xu LQ, Chen YD. Parasitic disease control and research in China. Beijing: Beijing Science and Technology Press; 2012.
3. WHO. 2015. Global technical strategy for malaria 2016–2030.
4. Chinese CDC. Technical protocol of malaria elimination in China. 2019.
5. Chinese CDC. Infectious Disease Surveillance Report in China in 2018.
6. Chinese CDC. Infectious Disease Surveillance Report in China in 2017.
7. Chinese CDC. Infectious Disease Surveillance Report in China in 2016.
8. Chinese CDC. Infectious Disease Surveillance Report in China in 2015.
9. Chinese CDC. Infectious Disease Surveillance Report in China in 2014.
10. Chinese CDC. Infectious Disease Surveillance Report in China in 2013.
11. Chinese CDC. Infectious Disease Surveillance Report in China in 2012.
12. Chinese CDC. Infectious Disease Surveillance Report in China in 2011.
13. Li ZJ, Yang YC, Xiao N, et al. Malaria imported from Ghana by returning gold miners, China, 2013. Emerg Infect Dis. 2015;21:864–7.
14. Infection Disease Report, Chinese CDC. Analysis of imported malaria cluster from May to August, 2013 in Shanglin, Guangxi. Feb. 2014.

10 Ebola Virus Disease Risk and Control

Chao Li and Qun Li

Ebola virus disease (EVD) is an acute infectious disease caused by the Ebola virus. It was first discovered in Africa in 1976. So far, it has mainly occurred in the Democratic Republic of Congo (DRC), the Republic of the Congo, Uganda, Gabon, the Republic of Sudan, Guinea, Liberia, Sierra Leone, Nigeria, Cote d'Ivoire, South Africa, and other African countries. Imported or laboratory infections have been detected in several countries around the world.

Ebola virus (EBOV) is subdivided into five species: Zaire (EBOV-Z), Sudan (EBOV-S), Bundibugyo (EBOV-B), Tai Forest (EBOV-TF), and Reston (EBOV-R). The Bombali virus newly isolated from fruit bats in Sierra Leone in 2018 may be the sixth species of the Ebola virus [1]. Among them, EBOV-Z, EBOV-S, and EBOV-B are all highly lethal to human beings. So far, EBOV-TF has only caused one severe case, while EBOV-R is not pathogenic to human beings, and it is not clear whether the Bombali virus is pathogenic to human beings or animals.

Currently it is believed that fruit bats (Pteropodidae) are the natural reservoirs of the Ebola virus [2], with humans and nonhuman primates infected with the Ebola virus as the main source of outbreak. Direct contact is the main way of EVD transmission. People can get EVD through direct contact with the blood, body fluids, secretions, excreta, or contaminated items of an infected animal or a sick or dead person infected with the Ebola virus. Research shows that the Ebola virus can still be detected in the semen of some male EVD survivors 3 months after their recovery, indicating that the virus can be transmitted through sexual contact [3]. At present, there is no evidence of airborne transmission of the Ebola virus, but there is still a risk of aerosol transmission at close range [4]. Places with a high risk of infection are mainly medical institutions and patients' homes. Without strict protective

C. Li · Q. Li (✉)
Chinese Center for Disease Control and Prevention, Beijing, People's Republic of China
e-mail: liqun@chinacdc.cn

W. Yang (ed.), *Prevention and Control of Infectious Diseases in BRI Countries*, https://doi.org/10.1007/978-981-33-6958-0_10

measures, healthcare workers, patients' families, or other close contacts are susceptible to infection during the treatment, nursing, or handling of a sick or dead person infected with Ebola virus.

Since the Ebola outbreak in West Africa in 2014, the global Ebola research has become active. According to WHO [5], the recombinant vesicular stomatitis virus vector vaccine (rVSV-ZEBOV-GP) developed by the Merck Group has passed the evaluation of the European Medicines Agency (EMA) and is expected to be approved for marketing. The vaccine has previously been used in clinical trials in Guinea and in response to the Ebola outbreak in DRC. In addition, a variety of vaccines, including recombinant adenovirus vector vaccine (Ad26-ZEBOV, chAd3-EBO-Z) and modified vaccinia virus Ankara vector vaccine (MVA-BN-Filo), are in clinical trials [6]. In August 2019, after the midterm analysis of the existing safety and effectiveness data, WHO believes that REGN-EB3 and mAb-114 can reduce mortality in patients who have received treatment early [7].

Although no Ebola cases have been found, China has actively participated in the prevention and control of the global Ebola outbreak. During the Ebola outbreak in West Africa between 2014 and 2015, China provided assistance including cash and supplies to epidemic-stricken countries and international organizations, with a total value of US$120 million. More than 1200 Chinese medical personnel and public health experts had been sent to epidemic-stricken areas and neighboring countries to complete nearly 9000 sample tests, observe and treat over 900 cases, and train 13,000 local people in medical care and community-based prevention and control. This is the biggest international health deployment in China. Some of these supports were channeled/facilitated by the WHO.

10.1 Ebola Virus Disease Epidemic

10.1.1 Overview

Since its first discovery in 1976, 46 EVD outbreaks have been reported in 20 countries around the world, and in particular, in Africa. Among them, DRC reported the most outbreaks, or a total of 10 (22%), followed by Uganda, a total of 6 (13%). Among all the outbreaks, 24 (52%) resulted in more than 10 infections, all of which occurred in African countries, with the majority of imported and laboratory infections in countries outside Africa (see Table 10.1).

Table 10.1 Statistics of Ebola outbreaks (by year)

Country	Year	Virus species	Infections	Deaths	Fatality rate (%)
Sudan	1976	EBOV-S	284	151	53
DRC		EBOV-Z	318	280	88
UK		EBOV-S	1	0	–
DRC	1977	EBOV-Z	1	1	–
Sudan	1979	EBOV-S	34	22	65

Table 10.1 (continued)

Country	Year	Virus species	Infections	Deaths	Fatality rate (%)
United States	1989	EBOV-R	0[a]	0	–
Philippines	1989	EBOV-R	3 (inapparent infection)	0	–
United States	1990	EBOV-R	4 (inapparent infection)	0	–
Italy	1992	EBOV-R	0[a]	0	–
Cote d'Ivoire	1994	EBOV-TF	1	0	–
Gabon		EBOV-Z	52	31	60
DRC	1995	EBOV-Z	315	254	81
Russia	1996	EBOV-Z	1	1	100
South Africa		EBOV-Z	2	1	50
Philippines		EBOV-R	0[a]	0	–
United States		EBOV-R	0[a]	0	–
Gabon		EBOV-Z	31	21	68
Gabon		EBOV-Z	60	45	75
Uganda	2000	EBOV-S	425	224	53
Republic of the Congo	2001	EBOV-Z	59	44	75
Gabon		EBOV-Z	65	53	81
Republic of the Congo	2003	EBOV-Z	143	128	89
Republic of the Congo		EBOV-Z	35	29	83
Sudan	2004	EBOV-S	17	7	41
Russia		EBOV-Z	1	1	–
Republic of the Congo	2005	EBOV-Z	12	10	83
DRC	2007	EBOV-Z	264	187	71
Uganda		EBOV-B	131	42	32
Philippines	2008	EBOV-R	6 (inapparent infection)	0	–
DRC		EBOV-Z	32	15	47
Uganda	2011	EBOV-S	1	1	100
DRC	2012	EBOV-B	38[b]	13[b]	34
Uganda		EBOV-S	11[b]	4[b]	36
Uganda		EBOV-S	6[b]	3[b]	50
Guinea, Liberia, Sierra Leone	2014	EBOV-Z	28,610	11,308	39
DRC		EBOV-Z	69	49	71
Italy		EBOV-Z	1	0	–
Mali		EBOV-Z	8	6	75
Nigeria		EBOV-Z	20	8	40
Senegal		EBOV-Z	1	0	–
Spain		EBOV-Z	1	0	–
UK		EBOV-Z	1	0	–
United States		EBOV-Z	4	1	25
DRC	2017	EBOV-Z	8	4	50
DRC	2018	EBOV-Z	54	33	61
DRC, Uganda		EBOV-Z	[c]	[c]	[c]

[a]Only animal infection, no human infection was found
[b]Laboratory confirmed cases only
[c]The epidemic continues, with data as of November 11, 2019

10.1.2 Epidemic in "Belt and Road Initiative" (BRI) Countries

Of the 20 countries that have reported Ebola outbreaks, 15 have signed a BRI cooperation agreement with China, including 12 African countries (Uganda, the Republic of Congo, Gabon, Sudan, Guinea, Liberia, Sierra Leone, South Africa, Mali, Nigeria, Senegal, and Cote d'Ivoire), 2 European countries (Russia and Italy), and the Philippines in Asia (see Table 10.2). The details are as follows.

10.1.2.1 Uganda

Uganda has reported a total of six Ebola outbreaks. Only the first two were large-scale outbreaks, while the remaining four were sporadic or clustered outbreaks. The first outbreak occurred in 2000–2001, which was also the largest outbreak in the history of the country. The outbreak first appeared in Gulu in the northern region of the country, bordering Sudan, and then spread to Masindi and Mbarara. The virus species was EBOV-S. It caused a total of 425 infections, including 224 deaths, with a fatality rate of 53% [8].

The second outbreak occurred in 2007–2008 in Bundibugyo District, where EBOV-B was first detected. The ability of the virus to spread is similar to other Ebola virus species but is slightly less severe after infection. In this epidemic, 131 people were infected and 42 (32%) were killed [9].

Since then, there has been no major outbreak in Uganda. In 2011, a case of EVD was reported in Luwero. Thanks to the strong early prevention and control measures, no subsequent infection occurred [10]. In 2012, a small-scale clustered outbreak occurred in Kibaale District, which resulted in eleven infections and four deaths [11]. In the same year, another outbreak was reported in the country, involving Luwero, Jinja, and Nakasongola. A total of six infections, including three deaths [11], were reported. These three outbreaks occurred between 2011 and 2012, all

Table 10.2 Overview of EVD outbreaks in the BRI countries

Country	Outbreak(s)	Infection(s) reported
Uganda	6	557
Gabon	4	208
Republic of the Congo	4	249
Sudan	3	335
Philippines	3	0
Russia	2	2
Italy	2	1
Guinea	1	3811
Liberia	1	10,675
Sierra Leone	1	14,124
South Africa	1	2
Mali	1	8
Nigeria	1	20
Senegal	1	1
Cote d'Ivoire	1	1

were caused by EBOV-S. The latest outbreak occurred in 2019 and was caused by an EBOV-Z outbreak in DRC. So far, four imported cases, all deceased, have been reported [11].

10.1.2.2 Gabon

Gabon has reported a total of four Ebola outbreaks, all caused by EBOV-Z. The first outbreak occurred in 1994 and was mainly in several rainforest villages around Makakou. At first, the epidemic was mistaken for a yellow fever outbreak, but a retrospective investigation revealed that the characteristics of the epidemic were different, and it was later confirmed as an Ebola outbreak in 1995 [12]. In this epidemic, 51 people were infected and 31 killed, with a fatality rate of 61%.

The second outbreak occurred in the spring of 1996, only 40 km from the first epidemic area. The outbreak was triggered by the slaughtering of a dead chimpanzee by local residents, followed by the infection and a gradual spread to close contacts. In this epidemic, 31 people were infected and 21 killed, with a fatality rate of 68% [13]. A similar outbreak reappeared in Booué in the autumn that year, with a total of 60 infections and 45 deaths, with a fatality rate of 75% [13].

The last outbreak in Gabon occurred in 2001–2002, in the region bordering the Republic of Congo. It was also due to an epidemic between animals, followed by an outbreak caused by human hunting and contact with wild animals, which eventually resulted in 65 infections and 53 deaths, with a fatality rate of 81% [14].

10.1.2.3 Republic of the Congo

The Republic of the Congo has reported a total of four Ebola outbreaks, all caused by EBOV-Z. The first outbreak, the last in Gabon as described earlier, occurred in 2001, resulting in a total of 59 infections and 44 deaths, with a fatality rate of 75% [14].

In early 2003, the second EVD outbreak occurred in the western part of the country. It was also caused by hunting and contact with wild animals, followed by the infection, a gradual spread through close family contacts, and a small spread in local medical facilities. It resulted in 143 infections and 128 deaths, with a fatality rate of 89% [15]. In November of the same year, 35 infections and 29 deaths were reported in the same region, with a fatality rate of 83% [16].

In 2005, the country reported its last outbreak to date, still in the western rainforests of the country. The index cases were two hunters who fell ill and died. Later, through nursing and funeral attendance, the epidemic spread further, resulting in 12 infections and 10 deaths, with a fatality rate of 83% [17].

10.1.2.4 Sudan

Sudan has reported a total of three Ebola outbreaks, all caused by EBOV-S. After the first detection of the Ebola virus in DRC in 1976, Sudan reported its first outbreak in the same year, starting at a cotton mill in the south of the country. The epidemic gradually spread to medical institutions through close contact and caused an outbreak there. A total of 284 infections and 151 deaths were reported, with a fatality rate of 53% [18].

In 1979, a second outbreak occurred in the same region. It was first reported by a textile mill, suggesting a similar source of infection to the first outbreak. Later onset records showed that the main mode of transmission was still close family contact, which resulted in 34 infections and 22 deaths, with a fatality rate of 65% [19].

The last outbreak in Sudan occurred in 2004 in an area close to where the previous two outbreaks occurred. The first infected person hunted baboons in the forest and came into contact with meat from wild animals 5 days before the onset. The epidemic spread for four generations, resulting in a total of seventeen infections and seven deaths, with a fatality rate of 41% [20].

10.1.2.5 Philippines

In 1989, researchers in the United States discovered a new species of Ebola virus, which was later named EBOV-R, after a large number of deaths in macaques exported from the Philippines to Reston, VA. Subsequently, the Philippines Department of Agriculture carried out serum screening on local staff and found a total of three persons with positive serum antibodies but no symptoms [21, 22].

In 1996, EBOV-R was detected again by the United States in macaques imported from the Philippines. This time, no human infection was found [23].

In 2008, the Philippines reported respiratory syndrome in domestic pigs, and later EBOV-R was detected again in the laboratory, which was the first time that the virus was detected in pigs. After serum tests were carried out on farm workers, six of them were found to be positive for serum antibody, but none showed clinical symptoms [24, 25].

10.1.2.6 Russia

Russia has reported a total of two Ebola outbreaks, both caused by laboratory infections, in 1996 and 2004. The tests involved research on drugs for treating Ebola and on vaccines [26, 27].

10.1.2.7 Italy

Italy has reported a total of two Ebola outbreaks. The first one occurred in 1992 when the Ebola virus was detected in monkeys imported from the Philippines but no human infection was found [28]. The second one occurred during the EVD outbreak in West Africa in 2014. An Italian healthcare worker who contracted the disease while volunteering at an Ebola treatment center in Sierra Leone returned to Italy before the onset of symptoms, finally he was cured and discharged from hospital [29].

10.1.2.8 Guinea, Sierra Leone, and Liberia

In 2014, Guinea, Sierra Leone, and Liberia witnessed the largest EVD outbreak in history. The epidemic originated in Gueckedou of Guinea. By March, more than 100 cases had been reported. With effective control efforts, the epidemic seemed to be under control. However, after Sierra Leone reported the epidemic in May, it expanded rapidly and the number of reported cases increased dramatically. In June, the epidemic developed rapidly in Liberia, and then entered a period of rapid development, and cases were exported to Nigeria, Senegal, the United States, Spain, and other countries. By 2016, the epidemic had lasted for nearly 2 years, affecting more than 10 countries, causing 28,646 infections and 11,323 deaths, with a fatality rate of 40%. Among them, 3811 infections occurred in Guinea and 2543 died, with a fatality rate of 67%; 10,675 infections occurred in Liberia and 4809 died, with a fatality rate of 45%; 14,124 infections occurred in Sierra Leone and 3956 died, with a fatality rate of 28%.

10.1.2.9 South Africa

In 1996, South Africa reported its one and only EVD outbreak. A healthcare worker from Gabon traveled to South Africa and was exposed because of his treatment of Ebola cases. He developed symptoms in South Africa and was cured. During the treatment, one nurse became infected and died later [30].

10.1.2.10 Cote d'Ivoire

In 1994, a large number of chimpanzees died in the Tai Forest of Cote d'Ivoire, and a researcher fell ill after performing an autopsy on the dead wild animals. During subsequent treatment and diagnosis, a new species of Ebola virus was discovered and later named EBOV-TF. The case was eventually cured, and it was the only outbreak caused by the EBOV-TF [31].

10.1.2.11 Mali, Nigeria, and Senegal

The EVD outbreaks in the three countries were all caused by the Ebola epidemic in West Africa in 2014, which only caused small-scale epidemic in Mali and Nigeria, and were quickly brought under control.

10.2 EVD Risk and Principles of Prevention and Control

10.2.1 EVD Risk

Currently it is believed that fruit bats (Pteropodidae), especially *Hypsignathus monstrosus*, *Epomops franqueti*, and *Myonycteris torquata*, are the natural reservoirs of Ebola virus [2]. These three fruit bats are widely distributed in Africa, so is the Ebola virus in nature. At the same time, people's lifestyles, living, and eating habits in Africa, as well as economic drivers and other factors lead to frequent contact between people and wild animals. Previous EVD outbreaks have proved that human killing, flaying of, and contact with wild animals are the main causes of the epidemic. Now that the source of infection continues to exist and the pathway of transmission cannot be blocked, human infections with the Ebola virus will continue to appear in Africa in the future.

It has been proved that the close contact at home and in medical facilities is the main cause of the spread of an epidemic, while some traditional cultures [32], customs [33], and benighted prejudices in Africa are the main driving factors for the further spread of epidemic. Besides, advances in transport also facilitate the mobility of infected people, thus promoting the spread of the disease from remote areas to and between cities. Therefore, once human infection cases occur, it is difficult to avoid small-scale clustered outbreaks in families or healthcare facilities, and it is impossible to rule out the possibility that the epidemic will spread to cities or even cause large-scale outbreaks across regions or countries.

For countries outside Africa, except for the risk of accidental laboratory infection, there is little risk of locally sourced outbreaks. However, in the process of globalization, international mobility is increasing. In particular, the "Belt and Road Initiative" proposed by China will further strengthen exchanges, cooperation, and trade among participating countries, so there is a risk of importing the Ebola virus disease. However, with the increasing attention of the international community to EVB epidemic, the accumulation of experience in dealing with it, and the gradual enrichment of response tools, even a large-scale outbreak (e.g., the outbreak in DRC in 2018) may only increase the risk of imported cases from a neighboring country, with an extremely low risk of reemergence of long-distance cross-country transmission.

10.2.2 Principles of EVD Prevention and Control

10.2.2.1 Reduce the Risk of Epidemic

As stated earlier, EVD, as a natural focus disease, is mainly caused by human killing, flaying of, and contact with wild animals. Therefore, changing human behavior can effectively reduce the incidence of infectious diseases. This mainly requires extensive social mobilization, publicity, and education to raise awareness and improve the preparedness of EVD. For example, reduce contact with wild animals, wear gloves when necessary, and do not eat raw animal products.

10.2.2.2 Early Detection of Outbreak

Most Ebola outbreaks are found in the form of clusters of epidemic or large-scale outbreaks, indicating that it is difficult to detect and identify early cases of infection. It is mainly because of inadequate surveillance capacity, local religious beliefs, and customs. When beliefs, customs, and other objective factors are difficult to change, it is crucial to improve the existing surveillance system and the regional capacity for Ebola surveillance and early identification. The earlier the outbreak is identified, the more conducive it is for the prevention and control work, and the lower the scope of the epidemic will be.

10.2.2.3 Isolate Patients, Follow Up, and Manage Close Contacts

Ebola virus is mainly spread by contact. Research shows that its basic reproduction number (R_0) is 1.33–2.7 [34–36], indicating that once human infection occurs, without timely and effective isolation, it is inevitable that the second generation of cases will occur, followed by small-scale clusters of the epidemic, or even large-scale outbreaks. However, EVD is not contagious during the incubation period, which clearly buys time for the early management of the epidemic. The risk of further spread can be effectively reduced if patients are treated in isolation early in the outbreak and all contacts are placed under medical observation.

10.2.2.4 Improve Public Cooperation in the Implementation of Prevention and Control Measures

During the EVD outbreak in West Africa in 2014, some communities misunderstood the public health intervention measures or the prevention and control measures offended with local religious beliefs or customs. As a result, they refused to cooperate. For example, there was a contradiction between the safe and dignified burial (SDB) and the traditional funeral customs, which was the cause for further expansion of the epidemic. Therefore, extensive social mobilization and health education are required, especially for religious or community leaders, which is conducive to the implementation of prevention and control measures.

10.3 Case Study

EVD Outbreak in West Africa

1. Overview

In early December 2013, Gueckedou in southern Guinea, Africa, experienced a cluster of mysterious disease cases with high fatality rates. They were characterized by fever, severe diarrhea, and vomiting, followed by similar cases in Macenta and Kissidougou (from December 2013 to March 2014, about 111 clinically suspected cases, including 79 deaths, occurred in these three prefectures). On March 10, 2014, public health institutions of Macenta and Kissidougou reported the outbreak of the unexplained disease to the Ministry of Health and Public Hygiene of Guinea. Two days later, the Ministry also informed the local Médecins Sans Frontières (MSF) of the epidemic. On March 18, MSF in Europe sent an investigation team to Macenta for epidemiological investigation and sent specimens of suspected cases to P4 laboratories in Lyon, France and Hamburg, Germany for detection. Three strains of the virus were isolated from 20 specimens of patients. Gene sequencing showed that it was EBOV-Z.

On March 22, 2014, WHO confirmed and announced an EVD outbreak in Guinea. As of March 27, 2014, more than 100 infections and 66 deaths had been reported. After that, the development of the epidemic was relatively slow and even seemed to be controlled. However, after WHO announced the outbreak in Sierra Leone in late May, the number of reported cases increased dramatically. In mid-June 2014, WHO announced a second wave of epidemic in Liberia, which spread rapidly, and the epidemic in the three countries in West Africa entered a period of rapid development, with a sharp rise in reported cases. Later, the total number of cases reported in Liberia and Sierra

Leone exceeded that in Guinea, and the epidemic spread to countries such as Senegal and Nigeria as a result of case exports.

As of March 27, 2016, the EVD outbreak affected 10 countries in total, among which the three countries in West Africa (Liberia, Sierra Leone, and Nigeria) were the most affected, with 28,646 infections and 11,323 deaths reported, with a fatality rate of 40%.

This outbreak, with the longest duration, the widest spread, and the highest number of reported cases since the discovery of the Ebola virus in 1976, was also the first EVD outbreak reported in West Africa.

2. Response

As the EVD outbreak continued, Guinea, Libya, and Sierra Leone were largely out of control. The intervention and control of the epidemic could not be completed independently by a single country or organization, rather, it required cooperation between countries and regions, as well as the full support of the international community. At the same time, comprehensive intervention measures were also carried out under the coordination of relevant United Nations agencies, including increasing medical facilities, improving the number and skills of healthcare workers, ensuring the treatment of patients in isolation, implementing the management of close contacts, strengthening harmless treatment of carcasses, reinforcing border inspection and quarantine, carrying out community health education, raising funds, etc.

In general, the response can be divided into three phases, including:

2.1 The phase of rapid scaling up of response activities. During Phase 1 (August–December 2014), as the epidemic dramatically worsened, WHO and its partners rapidly scaled up their response activities, including increasing Ebola treatment centers and beds, rapidly hiring and training teams to bury bodies in a safe and dignified manner, and strengthening capacity for social mobilization. During this period, the United Nations Mission for Ebola Emergency Response (UNMEER) was established.

2.2 Phase of capacity improvement. In January 2015, WHO and its partners entered Phase 2 (January–July 2015). The focus of this phase was to improve case detection capacity, improve the capacity to follow-up contacts, and improve community participation.

Thanks to these efforts and the start of Ebola vaccine trials in Guinea, the outbreak was basically brought under control and the number of Ebola cases and deaths dropped to single digits. WHO stressed that Guinea, Liberia, and Sierra Leone may be at risk of more small-scale Ebola outbreaks later due to the gradual elimination of the virus from survivors, and effective surveillance and response are still needed.

2.3 Phase of Ebola virus transmission blocking. In August 2015, WHO and its partners entered Phase 3 (August 2015 to mid-2016) with the overall goal of breaking all remaining chains of transmission. For this purpose, several specific objectives have been set, including further rapid identification of all infections, deaths, and contacts, establishment and maintenance of safe triage and healthcare facilities, establishment of multidisciplinary rapid response teams at the regional and local levels in the three countries, encouraging individuals and communities to follow public health measures, carrying out local response activities led by chiefs and controlled by communities, promoting participation and support of Ebola survivors, and ending human-to-human transmission of Ebola among people and communities in affected countries.

3. Experience and Lessons Learned

Looking back on the whole process of the response to the epidemic, it can be concluded that the failure of response at the early stage of the epidemic, including the late start of response in the three countries in West Africa, the slow response of the international community, as well as the delay in human and material assistance, thus missing the best time for epidemic control, is the root cause of its eventual evolution into an international public health concern. In addition, the lack of strong national leadership, the absence of effective organization and coordination in epidemic prevention and control, and the weak basic medical diagnosis are also the main causes of the spread of the epidemic.

The control of the epidemic in the later period mainly owes its success to the implementation of prevention and control in the following aspects: first, strict case management measures and isolation treatment for all suspected and confirmed cases; second, safe and dignified burial (SDB), with SDB teams set up to ensure the deceased can be handled reasonably and safely; third, strengthening surveillance and diagnosis, carrying out emergency surveillance, and improving the efficiency of laboratory diagnosis; fourth, active social mobilization, publicity and education, reaching out to communities and villages to raise public awareness of the disease, and joint efforts in prevention and control; fifth, strengthening personal protection, prevention and control of nosocomial infections, reducing the risk of further spread of the disease, and guaranteeing the strength of professional prevention and control teams.

Although the Ebola epidemic in West Africa has come to an end, the lessons and experiences are worth learning. From a macro perspective, the main revelation is that infectious disease respects no national borders. With the development of economy and culture, in the context of globalization, no country can be immune from the prevention and control of infectious diseases. An outbreak of infectious disease in any part of the world can quickly affect and impact any country and region. It is foreseeable that in the future, there will continue to be outbreaks of infectious disease or public health emergency, which will continue to pose a threat to people's health and safety, impact the political and economic development, and challenge the global public health. Therefore, in the future, only by accelerating the process of global health governance and coordinating global response can the occurrence of infectious diseases be effectively controlled and the impact of public health emergencies on the global economy and society be effectively reduced.

References

1. Goldstein T, Anthony SJ, Gbakima A, et al. The discovery of Bombali virus adds further support for bats as hosts of ebolaviruses. Nat Microbiol. 2018;3:1084–9.
2. Chunmei T, Huiyu L, Yuancong L. New advances in study of Ebola haemorrhagic fever [J]. Chin J New Clin Med. 2014;9:874–8.
3. Leroy EM, Epelboin A, Mondonge V, et al. Human Ebola outbreak resulting from direct exposure to fruit bats in Luebo, Democratic Republic of the Congo, 2007[J]. Vector Borne Zoonotic Dis. 2009;9(6):723–8.
4. Leffel EK, Reed DS. Marburg and Ebola viruses as aerosol threats. Biosecur Bioterror 2004;2(3):186–1191.
5. World Health Organization. Major milestone for WHO-supported Ebola vaccine. https://www.who.int/news-room/detail/18-10-2019-major-milestone-for-who-supported-ebola-vaccine.
6. Yves L, Lane C, Piot P, et al. Prevention of Ebola virus disease through vaccination: where we are in 2018. Lancet. 2018;392:787–90.
7. World Health Organization. Update on Ebola drug trial: two strong performers identified. https://www.who.int/news-room/detail/11-08-2019-update-on-ebola-drug-trial-two-strong-performers-identified.
8. Okware SI, Omaswa FG, Zaramba S, et al. An outbreak of Ebola in Uganda external icon. Tropical Med Int Health. 2002;7(12):1068–75.
9. MacNeil A, Farnon EC, Morgan OW, et al. Filovirus outbreak detection and surveillance: lessons from Bundibugyo. J Infect Dis. 2011;204:S761–7.
10. Shoemaker T, MacNeil A, Balinandi S, et al. Reemerging Sudan Ebola virus disease in Uganda, 2011. Emerg Infect Dis. 2012;18(9):1480–3.
11. Albarino CG, Shoemaker T, Khristova ML, et al. Genomic analysis of filoviruses associated with four viral hemorrhagic fever outbreaks in Uganda and the Democratic Republic of the Congo in 2012. Virology. 2013;442(2):97–100.
12. Milleliri JM, Tévi-Benissan C, Baize S, et al. Aspects épidémiologiques et réflexions sur les mesures de contrôle. Bull Soc Pathol Exot. 2004;97(3):199–205.
13. Georges AJ, Leroy EM, Renaud AA, et al. Ebola hemorrhagic fever outbreaks in Gabon, 1994–1997: epidemiologic and health control issues. J Infect Dis. 1999;179:S65–75.
14. World Health Organization. Outbreak(s) of Ebola haemorrhagic fever, Congo and Gabon October 2001–July 2002. Wkly Epidemiol Rep. 2003;78(26):223–5.
15. Formenty P, Libama F, Epelboin A, et al. Outbreak of Ebola hemorrhagic fever in the Republic of the Congo, 2003: a new strategy? Méd Trop (Marseille). 2003;63(3):291–5.
16. World Health Organization. Ebola haemorrhagic fever in the Republic of the Congo—Update 6. Wkly Epidemiol Rec. 2004;6.
17. Nkoghe D, Kone ML, Yada A, Leroy EA. Limited outbreak of Ebola haemorrhagic fever in Etoumbi, Republic of the Congo, 2005. Trans R Soc Trop Med Hyg. 2011;105:466–72.
18. World Health Organization. Ebola haemorrhagic fever in Sudan, 1976. Report of a WHO/International Study Team. Bull World Health Organ. 1978;56(2):247–70.
19. Baron RC, McCormick JB, Zubeir OA. Ebola virus disease in Southern Sudan: hospital dissemination and intrafamilial spread. Bull World Health Organ. 1983;61(6):997–1003.
20. World Health Organization. Outbreak of Ebola haemorrhagic fever in Yambio, South Sudan, April–June 2004. Wkly Epidemiol Rec. 2005;80(43):370–5.
21. Hayes CG, Burans JP, Ksiazek TG, et al. Outbreak of fatal illness among captive macaques in the Philippines caused by an Ebola-related filovirus. Am J Trop Med Hyg. 1992;46(6):664–71.
22. Miranda ME, White ME, Dayrit MM, Hayes CG, Ksiazek TG, Burans JP. Seroepidemiological study of filovirus related to Ebola in the Philippines. Lancet. 1991;337:425–6.
23. Miranda ME, Ksiazek TG, Retuya TJ, et al. Epidemiology of Ebola (subtype Reston) virus in the Philippines, 1996. J Infect Dis. 1999;179(suppl 1):S115–9.
24. World Health Organization. Ebola Reston in pigs and humans, Philippines. Wkly Epidemiol Rec. 2009;84(7):49–50.

25. Barrette RW, Metwally SA, Rowland JM, et al. Discovery of swine as a host for the Reston Ebola virus. Science. 2009;325:204–6.
26. Borisevich IV, Markin VA, Firsova IV, et al. Hemorrhagic (Marburg, Ebola, Lassa, and Bolivian) fevers: epidemiology, clinical pictures, and treatment. Voprosy Virusologii—Problem Virol (Moscow). 2006;51(5):8–16. [Russian].
27. Akinfeyeva LA, Aksyonova OI, Vasilyevich IV, et al. A case of Ebola hemorrhagic fever. Infektsionnye Bolezni (Moscow). 2005;3(1):85–8. [Russian].
28. World Health Organization. Viral haemorrhagic fever in imported monkeys. Wkly Epidemiol Rec. 1992;67(24):183.
29. World Health Organization. Ebola virus disease—Italy. Disease Outbreak News. 13 May 2015.
30. World Health Organization. Ebola haemorrhagic fever—South Africa. Wkly Epidemiol Rec. 1996;71(47):359.
31. Le Guenno B, Formenty P, Wyers M, et al. Isolation and partial characterisation of a new strain of Ebola virus. Lancet. 1995;345:1271–4.
32. Formenty P, Leroy EM, Epelboin A, et al. Detection of Ebola virus in oral fluid specimens during outbreaks of Ebola virus hemorrhagic fever in the Republic of the Congo. Clin Infect Dis 2006;42:1521–1521526.
33. Hilde DC. Struggling to contain the Ebola epidemic in West Africa. 2014. http://www.doctorswithoutborders.org/news-stories/voice-field/strugglingcontain-ebola-epidemic-west-africa.
34. Halparin C, Aranda S. Why Ebola patients are rejecting care. http://www.nytimes.com/video/world/africa/100000003019972/why-ebola-patientsare-rejecting-care.html.
35. Lekone PE, Finkenstadt BF. Statistical inference in A stochastic epidemic SEIR model with control intervention: Ebola as a case study. Biometrics. 2006;62:1170–7.
36. Pigott DM, Golding N, Mylne A, et al. Mapping the zoonotic niche of Ebola virus disease in Africa. elife. 2014;3:e04395.

Risk and Prevention of Middle East Respiratory Syndrome (MERS)

11

Yali Wang and Qun Li

Middle East respiratory syndrome (MERS), is a febrile respiratory disease caused by a new type of coronavirus discovered in September 2012 [1]. On May 23, 2013, the World Health Organization (WHO) named this new type of coronavirus as the Middle East respiratory syndrome coronavirus (MERS-CoV), and named the infection caused by MERS-CoV as MERS [2, 3].

11.1 ERS Outbreaks in the "Belt and Road Initiative" (BRI) Countries

Since the discovery of MERS in September 2012, as of September 30, 2019, WHO had announced 2468 confirmed cases, including 851 deaths, with a fatality rate of 34% [4]. The cases were distributed in 27 countries, including 11 in the Middle East (Saudi Arabia, UAE, Qatar, Jordan, Oman, Kuwait, Yemen, Egypt, Iran, Lebanon, Bahrain), 8 in Europe (Italy, France, Germany, UK, Greece, the Netherlands, Austria, Turkey), 5 in Asia (Malaysia, Philippines, South Korea, China, Thailand), 2 in Africa (Tunisia, Algeria), and 1 in North America (the United States). See Table 11.1 for details. Imported cases occurred in 14 countries in Europe, Asia, Africa, and North America. Of the reported cases globally, 84% occurred in Saudi Arabia (2077 cases) [4].

There are cases exported from Saudi Arabia, UAE, Qatar, Jordan, Oman, South Korea, etc., to other countries. In all outbreaks reported from countries outside the Middle East, all primary cases had a history of travel to or residence in the Middle

Y. Wang · Q. Li (✉)
Chinese Center for Disease Control and Prevention, Beijing, People's Republic of China
e-mail: liqun@chinacdc.cn

W. Yang (ed.), *Prevention and Control of Infectious Diseases in BRI Countries*,
https://doi.org/10.1007/978-981-33-6958-0_11

Table 11.1 MERS cases reported globally

Country	2012	2013	2014	2015	2016	2017	2018	2019	Total
Saudi Arabia	5	136	679	453	231	245	154	174	2077
UAE	0	12	57	7	3	7	1	1	88
Qatar	0	7	2	4	3	3			19
Jordan	2	0	10	16					28
Oman	0	1	1	4	2	2	1	13	24
Kuwait	0	2	1	1					4
Yemen	0	0	1	0					1
Egypt	0	0	1	0					1
Iran	0	0	5	1					6
Lebanon	0	0	1	0		1			2
Bahrain					1				1
South Korea	0	0	0	185			1		185
Italy	0	1	0	0					1
France	0	2	0	0					2
Germany	1	1	0	1					3
UK	1	3	0	0			1		5
Greece	0	0	1	0					1
The Netherlands	0	0	2	0					2
Austria	0	0	1	0	1				2
Turkey	0	0	1	0					1
United States	0	0	2	0					2
Tunisia	0	3	0	0					3
Algeria	0	0	2	0					2
China	0	0	0	1					1
Malaysia	0	0	1	0			1		2
Philippines	0	0	0	2					2
Thailand	0	0	0	1	2				3
Total	9	168	768	676	243	258	159	183	2468

East prior to the onset of symptoms or were epidemiologically linked to the imported cases from the Middle East. Among these countries, the United Kingdom, France, and Tunisia reported secondary cases, while South Korea reported secondary, third and fourth generation cases. In 2014–2015, there were several outbreaks of familial clustering and nosocomial infections in Saudi Arabia, UAE, South Korea, and other countries, but there were no reports of sustained transmission caused by the MERS virus in communities.

Among them, a total of 16 BRI countries reported MERS outbreak, including 13 West Asian countries and 3 ASEAN countries. Details are as follows:

1. Thirteen countries in Western Asia: Saudi Arabia, UAE, Qatar, Oman, Iran, Jordan, Lebanon, Yemen, Kuwait, Turkey, Greece, Egypt, and Bahrain.

(a) Saudi Arabia: Saudi Arabia was the first country suffering from MERS. On June 13, 2012, a 60-year-old man from Jeddah, Saudi Arabia was hospitalized, with symptoms of fever, cough, expectoration, and shortness of breath. It was the world's first case of MERS-CoV reported. From 2012 to late November 2019, Saudi Arabia reported 2077 confirmed MERS cases, the most in the world, or 84% of the world's total. In 2013–2015, a number of MERS outbreaks occurred in healthcare facilities or families in Saudi Arabia.

(b) UAE: So far, UAE has reported 88 confirmed MERS cases, the third highest after Saudi Arabia and South Korea.

(c) Qatar: So far, Qatar has reported a total of 19 confirmed MERS cases, with the last case developed on May 14, 2017, confirmed and reported on May 23. The case had frequent contact with camels in the 14 days before the onset of symptoms. No cases were reported in 2018 and 2019.

(d) Oman: Cases have been reported every year in Oman since 2013. So far, the country has reported a total of 24 confirmed MERS cases, with the most cases reported in 2019 (13 in total and linked to familial clusters).

(e) Iran: A total of six confirmed MERS cases were reported from Iran, including five in 2014 and one in 2015. The case reported in 2015 had close contact with two influenza-like cases returned from Umrah in the week before the onset.

(f) Jordan: A total of 28 confirmed MERS cases were reported from Jordan, including 2 in 2012, 10 in 2014, and 16 in 2015. No cases were reported in 2016–2019.

(g) Lebanon: On May 8, 2014, Lebanon reported its first confirmed MERS case. The case was a male, 60 years old, with underlying disease. From April 22, 2014, he successively developed symptoms of high fever, dyspnea, and dry cough. On April 27, he was diagnosed with pneumonia and hospitalized on April 30. On May 2, his specimen tested positive for MERS-CoV. He was cured and discharged from hospital on May 7, 2014. Epidemiological investigations showed that the case had no history of contact with dromedary camels, consumption of raw camel milk, or exposure to laboratory-confirmed cases in the 14 days before the onset of disease. However, the case had visited hospitals with MERS outbreaks in Saudi Arabia (8 weeks before the onset) and UAE (5 weeks before the onset). On June 16, 2017, another MERS case was confirmed, a 39-year-old male, who fell ill on June 8. He was a healthcare worker, but no MERS case was reported from the medical institution where he worked. He had no history of contact with camels, consumption of raw camel products, or exposure to confirmed MERS cases or patients suffering from respiratory disease. On June 11, he returned to Lebanon from Saudi Arabia without symptoms during the trip. On June 15, he developed gastrointestinal symptoms and an X-ray examination showed signs of pneumonia.

(h) Yemen: WHO announced the first MERS case in Yemen on May 7, 2014. The case, a 44-year-old male, developed symptoms on March 17, was admitted to hospital on March 22, 2014, and was transferred to a private hospital on March 29, 2014, where he was admitted to intensive care unit, complicated with renal failure. He died on March 31, diagnosed with hepatitis B. On May 5, his specimen tested positive for MERS-CoV in a laboratory in the United States. He had no history of travel or exposure to confirmed cases, but visited a camel farm and drank camel milk every week.
(i) Kuwait: On November 18, 2013, WHO announced the first laboratory-confirmed MERS case in Kuwait. A total of four confirmed MERS cases were reported from Kuwait, including two in 2013, one in 2014, and one in 2015. All the cases were male. The first three cases were close contacts of confirmed cases, and the last case reported on September 23, 2015 was 78 years old, with underlying disease. Epidemiological investigation showed that the case had a history of close contact with camels, with onset on September 8, confirmed on September 14, and died on September 19.
(j) Turkey: On April 24, 2014, it reported a male case, 42 years old, with onset on September 25, and died on October 11.
(k) Greece: On April 20, 2014, it reported a male case, 42 years old, with onset on April 17, and hospitalized on the same day.
(l) Egypt: On May 1, 2014, it reported a male case aged 27 who had lived in Riyadh, Saudi Arabia in the past 4 years. The case had contact with two confirmed cases (his uncle, who died on April 19) and his uncle's neighbor (who was receiving treatment in Jeddah). He had onset on April 22, returned to Egypt on April 25, and was laboratory confirmed on April 26.
(m) Bahrain: It reported the first case on April 25, 2016—a Saudi Arabian, male, 61 years old, with underlying disease. The case had onset on April 4, was confirmed on April 9, and died on April 12. He had a camel farm in Saudi Arabia, with a history of frequent contact with camels and drinking raw camel milk.

2. Three ASEAN countries: Malaysia, Thailand, and the Philippines.
   (a) Malaysia: The first MERS case, male, 54 years old, was reported on April 17, 2014. He had underlying diseases. From March 15 to 28, he made a pilgrimage to Jeddah, Saudi Arabia. On March 26, he went to a camel farm and drank camel milk. He had onset on April 4, 2014, was hospitalized on April 9, and died on April 13.

   On January 8, 2018, another case was reported. It was a male, 55 years old, with onset on December 24, 2017, and a history of contact with camels and drinking raw camel milk. He made a pilgrimage to Mecca, Saudi Arabia from December 13 to 23, 2017. During a visit to a camel farm in Riyadh on December 20, he contacted with dromedary camels (drinking unpasteurized camel milk and direct contact with camels). He developed symptoms on December 24 and was treated and hospitalized in Malaysia.
   (b) Thailand: On June 18, 2015, Thailand confirmed its first MERS case, imported from Oman, among travelers from the Middle East. WHO made an announcement on June 20, 2015. Two cases were confirmed on January 23

and July 28, 2016, respectively, which were also imported cases and from Oman and Kuwait, respectively.

(c) Philippines: Two MERS cases were reported from the Philippines, with the first one reported on February 13, 2015. The case, a 31-year-old female resident of Manila, was a healthcare worker working in Riyadh, Saudi Arabia. She flew to Manila with her family on February 1 and developed symptoms on January 26, 2105.

On July 8, 2015, WHO announced another case in the Philippines—a 36-year-old male, who traveled in Saudi Arabia between June 10 and 18 and stopped in Riyadh, Jeddah, and Dammam. He had a cough before his trip to Saudi Arabia. He left Saudi Arabia on June 18, stayed overnight in Dubai, UAE and arrived in Manila, the Philippines on June 19. From June 20 to 22, he was in Manila. Between June 23 and 24, he arrived in Malaysia from Manila, by way of Kuala Lumpur. On June 25, he returned to Manila from Malaysia, by way of Singapore. He had no symptoms during the trip. On June 30, he developed fever and cough. On July 2, he went to the hospital for treatment and his specimen was collected for laboratory test. He stayed at home on July 3. The test result was positive on July 4.

11.2 MERS Risk and Principles of Prevention and Control

11.2.1 Risk Assessment

WHO believes that the epidemiology, transmission patterns, clinical manifestations, and virus characteristics of MERS cases are consistent with those before. That is to say, MERS-CoV is a zoonosis virus that can infect humans directly or indirectly through direct or indirect contact with dromedary camel, with a high fatality rate. The virus has been shown to transmit from person to person. But so far, the limited, discontinuous human-to-human transmission observed has occurred primarily in healthcare facilities. Sporadic cases continue to be reported from Middle East countries and outbreaks can be imported into other countries outside the Middle East via human-to-human transmission, through contact with camels or camel products, in healthcare facilities, etc. [5].

11.2.2 Principles of Prevention and Control

1. WHO encourages all its member states to continue their surveillance for acute respiratory infections and to review carefully all unusual patterns.
2. Early identification, case management, and isolation, together with appropriate infection prevention and control measures, can prevent human-to-human transmission of MERS-CoV. As MERS-CoV infection is similar to other respiratory infections, the early symptoms are nonspecific. It is not always possible to identify patients with MERS-CoV infection early, and it is prone to nosocomial infection. Therefore, strict implementation of nosocomial infection prevention

and control measures is crucial to prevent the spread of MERS-CoV in healthcare facilities.

3. People should avoid close and unprotected contact with animals, particularly dromedary camels, when visiting farms, markets, or barn areas where the virus is known to be potentially circulating. General hygiene measures, such as regular hand washing before and after touching animals and avoiding contact with sick animals, should be adhered to.
4. Do not drink raw camel milk or camel urine, or eat meat that has not been properly cooked.
5. WHO does not advise special screening at points of entry with regard to MERS, nor does it currently recommend the application of any travel or trade restrictions [5].

11.3 Case Study

Management of Imported MERS Cases

1. Overview

On May 24, 2015, South Korea informed WHO of its first MERS case. Soon afterward, the case caused a continuous spread of MERS in Korean healthcare facilities. As of July 13, 2015, a total of 185 confirmed MERS cases (excluding one case imported to China), including 36 deaths, had been reported from South Korea. In addition to the first case, 12 cases caused secondary cases, of which 1 case caused 84 secondary cases [6]. The MERS outbreak in South Korea was the largest outside the Middle East. On May 29, 2015, China confirmed its first case of imported MERS from South Korea [7].

At 21:30 on May 27, 2015, the National Health and Family Planning Commission (NHFPC) received an informal notification from WHO Western Pacific that close contact of a confirmed MERS case in South Korea arrived in Huizhou, Guangdong Province by way of Hong Kong, and had developed fever (39.7 °C). After receiving the notification, the public health authorities promptly carried out case isolation treatment, epidemiological investigation, specimen collection and laboratory testing, close contact follow-up and management, and the implementation of nosocomial infection prevention and control measures. The case was discharged from hospital on June 26, 2015, and returned to South Korea. All 75 close contacts underwent 14 days of isolation for medical observation and no spread happened. The emergency was over.

2. Prevention and Control Practices

1. Implementing multisectoral prevention and control. On the basis of the coordination mechanism for dealing with epidemics established in 2012,

on June 9, 2015, NHFPC led the establishment of the multisectoral prevention and control mechanism that involved 17 ministries and commissions and released a corresponding work program to clarify responsibilities and strengthen information communication and coordination. Knowing a potential outbreak of imported epidemic in China, NHFPC organized relevant ministries and commissions to carry out joint supervision and inspection on epidemic prevention and control in Beijing, Shandong, Guangdong, Shanghai, Liaoning, Jilin, Gansu, and Xinjiang, so as to ensure that all prevention and control measures for MERS were fully implemented.

2. Responding rapidly to effectively prevent transmission in China. After receiving the information from WHO on the evening of May 27, it took just over 2 h to track down the male patient from South Korean and find out his movement path. He was then treated in isolation. At the same time, epidemiological investigation, specimen collection and laboratory testing, close contact follow-up and management, and nosocomial infection prevention and control measures were promptly carried out. After expert consultation organized by NHFPC on September 29, the case was confirmed as the first imported MERS case of China. On May 4, all 75 close contacts were tracked down and isolated for medical observation, which effectively prevented the potential spread in China.
3. Strengthening publicity, education, and public opinion guidance. While releasing epidemic information to the public in a timely, open, and transparent manner, the public health authorities actively carried out publicity and education on MERS prevention and control, guided the public to respond rationally and objectively, strengthened public opinion monitoring, and dispelled rumors in time.
4. Guiding the epidemic prevention and control among key populations, such as tourists and pilgrims to affected countries. The State Administration for Religious Affairs, NHFPC, AQSIQ, and other ministries and commissions issued emergency notices to guide epidemic prevention and control among pilgrims returned from Saudi Arabia. The health departments, together with tourism and other departments, guided the publicity and education of epidemic prevention and control knowledge for tourists and migrant workers in affected countries.
5. Strengthening international cooperation and exchanges. The Ministry of Foreign Affairs and NHFPC strengthened communication with WHO to keep abreast of the MERS situation and technical information on prevention and control, coordinated with South Korea for the latter to timely inform the progress of its epidemic prevention and control, and actively treated a Chinese citizen infected in South Korea (a female surnamed Jin, born in 1951, Jilin City, Jilin Province, cured and discharged from hospital on June 22). At the same time, NHFPC repeatedly expressed its willing-

ness to provide necessary help to South Korea. Feng Zijian, Deputy Director of China CDC, participated in the WHO-South Korea mission as an observer to communicate and guide the country's response to the MERS epidemic.

3. Experience and Lessons Learned

The SARS epidemic in 2003 was a "baptism" for China's public health emergency response system. The painful lessons greatly promoted the reconstruction and improvement of China's public health system [8], especially in recent years, in its response to emerging infectious diseases such as *Streptococcus suis*, hand, foot, and mouth disease, severe fever with thrombocytopenia syndrome, influenza A (H1N1), wild polio, human infection with H7N9 avian influenza, EVD, and so on. China's emergency response mechanism has been further improved, capabilities of infectious disease surveillance and laboratory testing continuously enhanced, the response mechanism of multisectoral prevention and control gradually strengthened, and the ability to prevent, control, and respond to infectious diseases, especially emerging infectious diseases, greatly improved. A timely, orderly, effective, and unhurried response can be achieved in the face of infectious diseases that may occur at any time. The South Korean Government's ineffective early warning, delayed response measures, and poor public information channels not only led to the MERS outbreak in the country, but also greatly affected the public's confidence in the government [8, 9]. In contrast, China has paid close attention to and prepared for an emergency since the discovery of a new SARS-like coronavirus in the Middle East in April 2012, including launching the multisectoral prevention and control mechanism, releasing prevention and control guidelines, preparing detection reagents, carrying out risk assessment, targeted training and drills [10]. The successful response to the imported MERS case shows that "we are quite experienced in disease prevention and control" [11], and we are fully capable of controlling this disease.

WHO spoke highly of China's response to the first imported case of MERS-CoV. Dr. Bernhard Schwartlander, WHO's representative to China, said that China had a very good mechanism to deal with emergencies like this, including well-trained isolation of suspected cases and high-quality treatment. The successful response to the first case not only blocked the spread of MERS in China, which has been highly appraised by the international community, but also accumulated rich experience in prevention, control, and treatment during the response.

References

1. National Health and Family Planning Commission, PRC. Middle East Respiratory Syndrome (MERS) Diagnosis and Treatment (2015 Edition), 2015.
2. Bermingham A, Chand MA, Brown CS, et al. Severe respiratory illness caused by a novel coronavirus in a patient transferred to the United Kingdom from the Middle East, September 2012. Euro Surveill. 2012;17(40):20290.
3. World Health Organization. Novel Coronavirus Infection Update, Middle East Respiratory Syndrome Coronavirus [2013-5-23] [EB/OL]. http://www.who.int/csr/don/2013-05-23-ncov/en/.
4. World Health Organization. MERS Situation Update, September 2019 [EB/OL]. http://applications.emro.who.int/docs/EMROPub-MERS-SEP-2019-EN.pdf?ua=1&ua=1.
5. World Health Organization. Disease Outbreak News, Middle East Respiratory Syndrome Coronavirus (MERS-CoV)-UAE [2019-10-31] [EB/OL]. https://www.who.int/csr/don/31-october-2019-mers-the-united-arab-emirates/en/.
6. Nijuan X, Dan L, Guangxu A, et al. Epidemiological features of Middle East respiratory syndrome in South Korea in 2015. Chin J Epidemiol. 2015;36(8):836–41.
7. Wu J, Yi L, Zou L, et al. Imported case of MERS-CoV infection identified in China, May 2015: detection and lesson learned. Euro Surveill. 2015;20(24):pii: 21158.
8. Li Qun. MERS in South Korea—humans once again showing their "Achilles' heel". Chin J Epidemiol. 2015;36(8):777–8.
9. Guang Z. International prevention and control of Middle East Respiratory Syndrome (MERS) and Ebola Virus Disease in 2015. Int J Epidemiol Infect Dis. 2016;43(1):1–3.
10. Zijian F. Be prepared for Middle East Respiratory Syndrome (MERS). Beijing: China Hospital CEO; 2019. p. 86–7.
11. Guangzhou Daily. China has a strong response mechanism. June 2, 2015.

Schistosomiasis Risk and Prevention 12

Yingjun Qian and Xiaonong Zhou

Schistosomiasis, as one of the 20 Neglected Tropical Diseases (NTDs) according to the World Health Organization (WHO), is threatening millions of lives in endemic areas, especially in Africa [1–3]. Schistosomiasis is highly prevalent in many low- and mid-income countries. The road map for neglected tropical diseases 2021–2030 set targets for elimination schistosomiasis as a public health problem in all 78 endemic countries by 2030.

Human schistosomiasis, also called bilharzia, refers to a parasitic disease caused by any of the parasitic blood flukes of *Schistosoma* spp. People get infected when they use fresh water contaminated by eggs of schistosome through daily life, such as farming, fishing, swimming, washing clothes, and other activities. In total, six species of schistosomes are responsible for human infections, which are *Schistosoma haematobium, Schistosoma mansoni, Schistosoma japonicum, Schistosoma mekongi, Schistosoma intercalatum,* and *Schistosoma guineensis.* Among these, *S. haematobium and S. mansoni* are the dominating burden attributed to schistosomiasis, especially in sub-Saharan Africa. *S haematobium and S mansoni* occur in Africa, the Middle East, South America, and the Caribbean [4, 5], while *S japonicum* is localized to Asia, primarily the Philippines and China. The other species are more locally distributed [6]. Each species has a specific range of suitable freshwater snail to act as hosts, which determines the geographical distribution of the corresponding disease.

Y. Qian · X. Zhou (✉)
National Institute of Parasitic Diseases, China CDC, Shanghai, People's Republic of China
e-mail: zhouxn1@chinacdc.cn

W. Yang (ed.), *Prevention and Control of Infectious Diseases in BRI Countries*,
https://doi.org/10.1007/978-981-33-6958-0_12

Millions of infected people suffer from severe morbidity as a consequence of schistosomiasis. It can result in long-term, severe complications, such as intestinal, hepatic, bladder, and ureteric fibrosis, and bladder cancer as well. Schistosomiasis can cause profound negative effects on child development, outcome of pregnancy, and labor force. Growth retardation, weakness, impairment cognitive development, and increased risk of anemia in children infected with schistosoma can result in poor academic performance and hamper their potential [7, 8]. These negative outcomes in children add to the socioeconomic burden of the society. Except for *S haematobium*, which is the engine for urogenital schistosomiasis, the other schistosomiasis mainly affect human intestine and liver. In addition, it is important to know that female genital schistosomiasis, affecting over 56 million women in endemic areas, can cause considerable inequity, social exclusion, and stigma for women and girls.

12.1 Overview of Schistosomiasis in "Belt and Road" Countries

12.1.1 Epidemiological Situation

Schistosomiasis is prevalent in tropical and subtropical areas, especially in poor areas without adequate sanitation and lack of safe water supply. Globally, approximately 240 million people are infected by schistosomiasis, and over 700 million are in endemic areas. According to the WHO estimation, at least 90% of those requiring treatment for schistosomiasis live in Africa. However, the underestimate of the burden of the disease restricts control efforts in those areas, which in turn, further intensifies the threats in public health.

It is estimated that there are at least 290.8 million people who required preventive treatment for schistosomiasis in 2018, out of whom over 97.2 million were reported to have been treated [9]. Recent research showed that there were 207 million infections in the world, of which 93% occurred in Sub-Sahara Africa, with the largest number in Nigeria (29 million) followed by United Republic of Tanzania (19 million), and DRC and Ghana (15 million each) [10, 11].

12.1.1.1 Nigeria

Nigeria, with 20 million people requiring schistosomiasis treatment, is ranked highest among the countries of the world endemic for the disease [10]. Both intestinal and urinogenital schistosomiasis occur in Nigeria. Three species of *Schistosoma* can be found in Nigeria: *S. haematobium* in South, *S. mansoni* in North, and *S. intercalatum* is rarely or misdiagnosed for *S. haematobium* [12, 13]. Previous studies revealed the prevalence rates ranged between 14.2% and 91.4%. However, the exact level of prevalence of urinary schistosomiasis in Nigeria remains unknown. Information are cumulative by many scattered research output and there are no baseline data or nationwide surveys up to now. Urinary schistosomiasis accounts for at least 90% of all cases in Nigeria, indicating that the disease burden is mainly caused by urinary schistosomiasis [14]. Although with 74% coverage of mass drug administration (MDA), in Nigeria schistosomiasis appears to be a serious health problem. Prevalence in school children can be as high as 70%, and in population once thought not to be at a high-risk group, observed prevalence level is 20%. In some Southwestern part, prevalence appears to be ranging from 44.8% to 71.5% in endemic areas. MDA is the unique intervention to control schistosomiasis in Nigeria, but far from enough to sustain long-term achievements.

12.1.1.2 Tanzania

It was showed that following Nigeria, Tanzania ranks the second top number of schistosomiasis infection in sub-Saharan Africa [15]. The estimation was about 52% of the Tanzanian population, equal to 23 million were infected with schistosomiasis. Both intestinal and urogenital schistosomiasis are prevalent in this country. *S. mansoni* is focally distributed along large water bodies. It is highly ordinarily seen among both school children and adults. More recently, research indicates that even in the population of preschool aged children, schistosomiasis has been detected with heavy intensities.

12.1.1.3 Ghana

Schistosomiasis is prevalent in Ghana and the predominant control strategy is to reduce morbidity in children through annual MDA of praziquantel following WHO recommendations. Ghana has been implementing this strategy since 2007 for STH and 2008 for SCH. A recent study showed as high as 44.2% prevalence of *S. mansoni* and 11.9% of *S. haematobium* in the Greater Accra region, Ghana. In some areas, the prevalence of infection for *S. mansoni* reached 80.1% and 79.1% in school-age children and adults, respectively [14]. For *S. haematobium*, the prevalence was 35.9% and 34.8% in school-age children and adults, respectively. Another research used urine-CCA assay to test the prevalence and showed 90.5%, 87.9%, and 81.2% in 190 preschool-aged children [16]. Therefore, it is conceivable that both intestinal and urogenital schistosomiasis are prevalent in the country.

12.1.2 Control Progress

Currently, the key strategy for schistosomiasis control and elimination is to implement treatment, which is called preventive chemotherapy. Therefore, in many settings, the progress of schistosomiasis depends on the implementation of preventive chemotherapy.

According to the WHO report, it was estimated that 95.3 million populations were affected by schistosomiasis worldwide [17]. In 2018, approximately a number of 124.4 million school-aged children globally were in need of treatment for schistosomiasis, an index for 54.3% of all people globally. Of the 124.4 million, 76.2 million received treatment, showing the global coverage of 61.2%. In the world, a total of 34 countries reported to carry out schistosomiasis treatment in 2018 and the reporting rate was 65.4% [16]. Table 12.1 shows the global implementation of preventive chemotherapy in 2018.

Table 12.1 Population-based data on preventive chemotherapy for schistosomiasis in 2019 (Source: WHO)

Region	Country	SAC population requiring PC for SCH annually	Population requiring PC for SCH annually	Reported number of people treated	Age group	Reported number of SAC treated	National coverage (%)
AFR	Angola	4,068,555	7,089,384	1,116,928	SAC	1,116,928	15.75%
AFR	Benin	1,394,252	2,362,208	804,844	SAC	804,844	34.07%
AFR	Botswana	151,489	177,125				
AFR	Burkina Faso	2,170,725	3,286,767	2,924,740	SAC and adults	1,808,698	88.99%
AFR	Burundi	1,518,749	1,585,087	1,493,458	SAC	1,493,458	94.22%
AFR	Cameroon	3,124,677	5,402,652	5,173,178	SAC and adults	3,050,947	95.75%
AFR	Central African Republic	477,715	1,216,727	448,056	SAC	448,056	36.82%
AFR	Chad	2,331,865	3,891,239	1,543,409	SAC	1,543,409	39.66%
AFR	Congo	218,664	408,975				
AFR	Côte d’Ivoire	2,650,436	4,599,701	1,782,425	SAC and adults	1,419,714	38.75%
AFR	Democratic Republic of the Congo	11,189,444	15,513,369	7,562,926	SAC	7,562,926	48.75%
AFR	Equatorial Guinea	32,196	62,864				
AFR	Eritrea	228,485	417,622	383,072	SAC and adults	211,390	91.73%
AFR	Eswatini	282,396	402,727				
AFR	Ethiopia	7,513,321	14,016,869	5,002,918	SAC and adults	4,513,662	35.69%
AFR	Gabon	189,108	208,406				
AFR	Gambia	98,488	134,990				
AFR	Ghana	4,369,206	10,685,201	3,974,240	SAC	3,974,240	37.19%
AFR	Guinea	1,763,592	4,031,094				
AFR	Guinea-Bissau	430,700	439,899				
AFR	Kenya	1,924,082	3,519,321	545,263	SAC and adults	382,608	15.49%
AFR	Liberia	605,166	1,035,146	539,432	SAC	539,432	52.11%
AFR	Madagascar	4,319,747	10,210,974	2,842,764	SAC	2,842,764	27.84%
AFR	Malawi	4,216,093	9,194,638	4,784,184	SAC and adults	3,956,123	52.03%
AFR	Mali	3,461,508	6,049,294	4,064,696	SAC and adults	3,296,877	67.19%

AFR	Mauritania	382,778	826,827	213,171	SAC	213,171	25.78%
AFR	Mozambique	5,958,820	15,726,917	5,713,771	SAC	5,713,771	36.33%
AFR	Namibia	203,961	486,997				
AFR	Niger	2,607,881	6,262,985	6,254,428	SAC and adults	2,599,325	99.86%
AFR	Nigeria	17,133,694	25,811,970	21,061,922	SAC and adults	16,930,352	81.60%
AFR	Rwanda	1,623,922	2,652,896	1,242,667	SAC and adults	1,144,650	46.84%
AFR	Sao Tome and Principe	23,124	38,140	14,094	SAC	14,094	36.95%
AFR	Senegal	1,923,202	4,282,543	1,555,894	SAC and adults	1,458,350	36.33%
AFR	Sierra Leone	1,252,782	2,753,175	1,340,150	SAC and adults	1,051,150	48.68%
AFR	South Africa	2,623,952	5,603,448				
AFR	South Sudan	1,336,336	2,884,192	147,138	SAC	147,138	5.10%
AFR	Togo	1,203,304	2,464,417	407,848	SAC	407,848	16.55%
AFR	Uganda	5,573,009	12,274,035	3,417,779	SAC	3,417,779	27.85%
AFR	United Republic of Tanzania	6,576,725	14,874,954	4,260,600	SAC	4,260,600	28.64%
AFR	Zambia	3,040,896	4,756,368				
AFR	Zimbabwe	2,470,412	3,828,849				
AMR	Brazil	1,550,386	1,556,890				
AMR	Venezuela (Bolivarian Republic of)	63,940	63,940				
EMR	Egypt	3,722,983	6,894,411	6,894,411	SAC and adults	3,722,983	100.00%
EMR	Somalia	1,434,961	1,663,712				
EMR	Sudan	4,516,705	8,080,706	3,058,201	SAC and adults	2,483,677	37.85%
EMR	Yemen	3,305,807	3,943,893	3,104,097	SAC	3,104,097	78.71%
SEAR	Indonesia	5800	21,815	19,222	SAC and adults	4103	88.11%
WPR	Cambodia	40,005	108,227	89,908	SAC and adults	32,564	83.07%
WPR	China	No PC required	No PC required				
WPR	Lao People's Democratic Republic	28,780	112,614	90,963	SAC and adults	26,873	80.77%
WPR	Philippines	1,002,165	2,719,004	1,518,370	SAC and adults	559,638	55.84%

PC preventive chemotherapy, *SCH* schistosomiasis, *SAC* school-age children

A number of countries have carried out control programs for schistosomiasis at national level, such as China, the Philippines, Morocco, Brazil, Iran, Egypt, and Tunisia. In these countries, distribution of praziquantel was conducted at large scale. Result showed that transmission of schistosomiasis was significantly reduced in the countries. Some of them reached a low-endemicity status, while others were unable to consolidate their achievements, where the infection returned to preintervention levels [18, 19].

In total, there are altogether 78 countries where schistosomiasis is prevalent, of which 42 are in the WHO African Region [20]. Three additional countries and one territory can be added to the list for a comprehensive database. The additional countries and territories are as follows: Eritrea, Montserrat, South Sudan, and Djibouti [20]. In Asia, prevalence of schistosomiasis in all four endemic countries Cambodia, China, the Lao People's Democratic Republic, and the Philippines has declined significantly. China has shifted from MDAs to selective and targeted treatment. Cambodia and the Lao People's Democratic Republic sustained above 75% coverage with preventive chemotherapy among all school-aged children and adults in endemic villages. As a result, Cambodia, China, and the Lao People's Democratic Republic achieved the criteria for elimination of schistosomiasis as a public health problem by 2017. The Philippines continued to make efforts to improve MDA coverage nationwide [19].

Schistosomiasis has been successfully eliminated in Japan and Tunisia. Morocco and some Caribbean Islands countries have made significant progress on controlling the disease, while Brazil, China, and Egypt are taking steps toward elimination of the disease (Fig. 12.1) [7].

According to the 2021–2030 roadmap of NTD, schistosomiasis elimination as a public health problem is targeted for elimination in the WHO Eastern Mediterranean Region, the Caribbean, and the WHO Western Pacific Region [17].

Group	Countries and territories
Countries requiring preventive chemotherapy	African Region: Angola, Benin, Botswana, Burkina Faso, Burundi, Cameroon, Central African Republic, Chad, Congo, Cote d'Ivoire, Democratic Republic of the Congo, Equatorial Guinea, Eritrea, Ethiopia, Gabon, Gambia, Ghana, Guinea, Guinea-Bissau, Kenya, Liberia, Madagascar, Malawi, Mali, Mauritania, Mozambique, Namibia, Niger, Nigeria, Rwanda, Sao Tome and Principe, Senegal, Sierra Leone, Sierra Leone, South Africa, Swaziland, Togo, Uganda, United Republic of Tanzania, Zambia, Zimbabwe
	Region of the Americas: Brazil, Venezuela (Bolivarian Republic of)
	Eastern Mediterranean Region: Egypt, Somalia, South Sudan, Sudan, Yemen
	South-East Asia Region: Indonesia
	Western Pacific Region: Cambodia, China, Lao People's Democratic Reblic, Philippines
Countries requiring updating for planning and implementation purposes	Region of the Americas: Saint Lucia, Suriname
	Eastern Mediterranean Region: Iraq, Libya, Oman, Saudi Arabia, Syrian Arab Republic
Countries requiring evaluation in order to verify if interruption of transmission has been achived	African Region: Algeria Mauritius
	Redion of the Americas: Antigua, Dominican Republic, Guadeloupe, Martinique, Monterrat, puerto Rico
	Eastern Mediterranean Region: Djibouti, Iran (Islamic Republic of), Jordan, Lebanon, Morocco, Tunisia
	European Region: Turkey
	South-East Asia Redion: India, Thailand
	Western Pacific Redion: Japan, Malaysia

Fig. 12.1 Status of schistosomiasis endemic countries in the WHO regions

In the past decades, several countries have successfully implemented schistosomiasis control. Large-scale treatment was conducted in a number of countries, such as China, Egypt, Brazil, and Morocco, resulting in significant reduction in both infection and morbidity. After a successful vertical program in Brazil, the disease control program was devolved to local health services. In China, Egypt, and Morocco, programs were implemented through primary healthcare systems but with central direction for significant reduction or interruption of transmission. Few other countries have undertaken large-scale preventive chemotherapy for schistosomiasis, therefore, the goal to have regularly treated at least 75% of school-age children worldwide by 2010 has not been attained. The major impediment to schistosomiasis control is the limited access to praziquantel. Moreover, many endemic countries do not have public health infrastructure or necessary resources to implement schistosomiasis control. In WHO's African Region, no new cases of schistosomiasis have been detected in school-age children from Mauritius since 1991, indicating that the disease can be considered eliminated from it. Algeria is another country with no case reported. According to the WHO Regional Office for the Americas, there have been no cases of schistosomiasis reported from Antigua, the Dominican Republic, Guadeloupe, Martinique, Montserrat, and Puerto Rico. Several countries of WHO's Eastern Mediterranean Region seem to have interrupted schistosomiasis transmission, such as Jordan, the Islamic Republic of Iran, Morocco, and Tunisia. No cases have been reported in the past 50 years from Turkey in the WHO European Region. Only Japan and Malaysia in the Western Pacific Region seem to have eliminated schistosomiasis.

12.2 Schistosomiasis Risk and Control Principles

12.2.1 Schistosomiasis Risk

12.2.1.1 Sustained Risks in Local Schistosomiasis Transmission

12.2.1.1.1 Lack of Safe Water, Inadequate Sanitation, and Behavior

One of the risk factors is water contact in endemic areas where safe water supply, sanitation, and individual hygiene are inadequate in endemic settings. Clean water and hygiene are crucial for local people to prevent from contacting with infested water source. Good practices in personal hygiene are also helpful to avoid being infected. Although WHO set targets for safe water, sanitation, and hygiene [18], many authorities in sub-Saharan Africa are not dedicated to making available clean water sources for their communities, making it still hard to achieve [21–23].

12.2.1.1.2 Widely Distributed Snail Habitats

Schistosomiasis transmission relies on the presence of an appropriate freshwater snail host. The different schistosome species require their own specific snail host species in order to complete life cycles. For example, *Bulinus spp.* Snails are responsible for the transmission of *S. haematobium*, is transmitted by *Biomphalaria*, is the vector for *S. mansoni*, and the intermediate host of *S. japonicum* is *Oncomelania* snails. Snail colonization of local water habitats, whether rivers, streams, ponds, paddies, or ditches, sets the stage for schistosome transmission to humans [24].

12.2.1.1.3 Risk of Reinfection

Literature shows typical childhood infection/reinfection rates vary from 7% to 26% each year in areas endemic for *S. haematobium*, from 15% to 30% each year for *S. mansoni*, from 4% to 23% each year for *S. japonicum* [25]. The common reason why people get reinfected could be depicted because of the following factors, repeating routine behaviors in lack of access to acceptable water infrastructure, lack of knowledge, and/or risky attitudes and practices [26].

12.2.1.2 Risk of Imported Schistosomiasis Transmission

Population growth and movement is a major factor in schistosomiasis transmission to new areas. In none endemic areas and/or areas where schistosomiasis is eliminated, the risks of imported schistosomiasis and local transmission given that breeding sites present for appropriate snail vectors are undoubtedly steadily rising due to ever-increasing population inflows from endemic areas. In China, since 1970s when the program to aid African infrastructure construction began, imported cases with *S. mansoni* and/or *S. haematobium* infections have been continuously inspected in returners from Africa. As a result, the majority of infection were field workers diagnosed during checkups. Additionally, because of slight or even no clinical manifestations, infection with *S. mansoni* was often neglected by these migrant workers who rarely seek medical services. On the other hand, these non-specific symptoms easily led to missed diagnosis. Therefore, it is presumable that the real number of infections was far from those reported. It was reported that the imported schistosomiasis cases especially from Africa were widely distributed in China. A survey of 263 Chinese workers from Africa infected with *S. haematobium* showed a wide distribution in 17 provinces in China [22]. Another case was seen in eight European students infected with *Schistosoma* after several months stay with freshwater exposure history in Tanzania [27, 28].

12.2.2 Control Strategies

Preventive chemotherapy is referred to the distribution of safe medicines, either alone or in combination, to population groups at risk at a large scale. Preventive chemotherapy can be carried out at regular intervals targeting at decreasing morbidity and ultimately interrupt disease transmission. The WHO strategy of preventive chemotherapy by usage of anthelminthic drugs makes it possible to control schistosomiasis in poor and marginalized communities, alongside lymphatic filariasis, onchocerciasis, soil-transmitted helminthiasis, and trachoma [24]. Praziquantel has been safely co-administered with albendazole and ivermectin, in areas where these drugs have been used separately for preventive chemotherapy. However, in most African countries, preventive chemotherapy is the only control intervention and often applied in school-age children. For drug only, the inadequate supply of praziquantel and the insufficient distribution system also makes it difficult to carry out control programs. Schistosomiasis control is more of an integrated program than preventive chemotherapy only if the ultimate goal of elimination is to be met. The implementation of complementary interventions combined with preventive chemotherapy is strongly recommended by WHO.

12.2.2.1 Preventive Chemotherapy

The most rapid and cost-effective means to prevent and reduce the morbidity of schistosomiasis is chemotherapy with praziquantel [16, 29]. More than 90% of these people live in sub-Saharan Africa and require preventive chemotherapy. Most countries in sub-Saharan Africa endemic for schistosomiasis are not in a position to establish a country-wide elimination program due to high prevalence rates and transmission potential.

At present, preventive chemotherapy still remains the most important interventions in schistosomiasis control for morbidity control, transmission interruption, and disease elimination and eradication. When the prevalence is very high, preventive chemotherapy aims to reduce severe infections. In the transmission interruption stage, preventive chemotherapy should be expanded to the target population, and the frequency of treatment should be increased. In some cases, such as control of schistosomiasis japonica in China, due to its variety of animal reservoirs, it is key to treat the animals or to prevent them from contaminating the environment.

In practice, preventive chemotherapy interventions can be implemented as modalities, mass drug administration (MDA) referring to treat the entire population in an area, targeted chemotherapy which is implemented to specific risk groups, and selective chemotherapy, which means treatment to be conducted in all infected individuals living in an endemic area as a result of regular screening in a population [17].

12.2.2.2 Snail Control

With the adoption of resolution WHA65.21 by 65th World Health Assembly in 2012, the elimination of schistosomiasis where appropriate reshapes the global agenda of the schistosomiasis control community. Evidence showed that regular mollusciciding is likely to advance schistosomiasis elimination, particularly in high-risk areas. As a matter of fact, for many years snail control as the one of the key methods to control schistosomiasis has been implemented by molluscicides, and environmental and biological methods. While the attention and resources focused on preventive chemotherapy over the past two decades have yielded many benefits, the focus on chemotherapy in Africa has perhaps hindered the development of new approaches for snail control and, consequently, led to a general decline in global malacological expertise [25]. Snail control was successfully carried out to achieve schistosomiasis eradication in Morocco and Japan and it has been implemented in control program in Egypt and China. However, toxicity of the chemical to fish and other water-dwelling organisms should be attached great importance both ecologically and economically. Alternatives to chemical-based molluscicides include the use of plant-based derivatives and biological control with snail competitors [30].

12.2.2.3 Sanitation Improvement and Safe Water Supply

Access to and use of clean, safe water and improved sanitation are proved to be essential in preventing infection in endemic areas. Also, it is important to point out that better access to safe water and sanitation does not necessarily intensify transmission control and/or interruption because of various water source for difference purposes. For instance, latrines may impact on the transmission of intestinal schistosomiasis, but they may not have same impacts on that of urogenital schistosomiasis. While preventive chemotherapy can be used to produce immediate impacts in reducing disease burden, such interventions in sanitation and access to safe water sustain effects and achievements can further decrease infection rate and interrupt transmission. Also, clean water and hygiene are essential for provision of appropriate care and rehabilitation services for those affected by residual morbidities and chronic disabilities [26].

12.2.2.4 Hygiene Education

Since contacting open water bodies contaminated with excreta of infected people in most rural settings is inevitable, behavior change and health education of the population is necessary. Comprehensive health education activities for all population to guide behavioral change, especially avoid water contact is in need. Health education to both children and adults has been proved to impact health-seeking behavior, which may reduce prevalence of infection.

Intensified efforts of behavior change need to be made to the population on the risk of infection and transmission regarding waste elimination and personal exposure to open water sources. Residents in endemic areas need to be encouraged to reduce water contact for the purpose of transmission reduction [31]. It is necessary that health education must be carried out in consideration of local settings, and should be practiced through interaction rather than one-direction instructions. Cultural sensitivity is a sensitive component when health education tools are designed and developed.

12.2.2.5 Disease Surveillance

Surveillance is always a key component of schistosomiasis control and elimination. In control stage, when the goal is to lower the heavy disease burden, routine surveillance is carried out to dynamically monitor the reduction in infections, which serves as a good tool for intervention guideline and effect assessment of control activities. All transmission foci should be identified, and appropriate interventions undertaken. When the goal is disease elimination, surveillance should be gradually strengthened in all previously endemic areas for the purpose of case detection and quick response to prevent reintroduction from endemic areas. Sentinel sites should be systematically set up for routine disease surveillance, as one part of the health systems. Surveillance is an essential component of an elimination program so that each transmission foci is identified to consolidate achievements. For example, schistosomiasis is notifiable in China and each case is promptly reported to the national health system in 24 h. Nevertheless, other routine interventions, such as snail control, health education, and sanitation improvement still work as components of an elimination program.

12.3 Case Study

Schistosomiasis Control in China

In China, the first case was recorded by an American doctor in Changde, Hunan province, in 1905. However, the disease carries a long history in China which could be dated back to over 2000 years ago when eggs of Schistosoma japonicum were discovered in the Changsha Mawangdui tumulus [27]. Only schistosomiasis japonica is endemic in China and Oncomelania hupensis is the unique intermediate host.

Schistosomiasis in China was of high prevalence in 12 provinces (municipality and autonomous region) along south of the Yangtze River. The highest estimation of patients was 12 million in the 1950s. Since then, schistosomiasis control has been always a high priority led by the Chinese central government. From 1950s till now, national strategies on schistosomiasis control changed from disease elimination through snail control focused to morbidity control by preventive chemotherapy, and now integrated control with an emphasis on management of infection source. In addition, as domestic animals play an important role as reservoirs, livestock, especially buffaloes, were also treated at the same time.

By the end of 2019, 5 of the 12 provinces (municipality and autonomous region) continued to consolidate the achievements of schistosomiasis elimination, one achieved transmission interruption, one newly achieved the standard of transmission interruption, and the rest of the five maintained transmission control. According to the 2019 national report [28], a total of 327,475 individuals received stool examinations and five were positive, of which one was acute schistosomiasis. These significant achievements are attributed to the strong political commitment, the uninterrupted implementation of the cross-sectional national control program led by the government, the scientific research and development of new tools and technology, and the continuous surveillance activities. Research programs pertaining to schistosomiasis were listed as key programs in the ministries of health, agriculture, and water resources. By the end of 2011, except one national institute, there had been 365 agencies for schistosomiasis control in seven provinces. Among them, 282 were responsible for schistosomiasis control, and the others were in charge of prevention and clinical case management. New technologies such as remote sensing, geographical information system, predictive statistical modelling, and xeno-monitoring based on loop-mediated isothermal amplification techniques are also adopted. These activities provide basic information for decision-makers and facilitate the assessment of the achievements obtained through decades of efforts [2].

China-Zanzibar Schistosomiasis Control Project

With more than 70 years of schistosomiasis control activities, China have gained a great success on the disease control, and the experience can be shared to other countries. China also expressed its willingness to cooperate with

African countries in the field of public health. On May 21, 2014, China, Zanzibar, and WHO jointly signed a memorandum of understanding on cooperation in schistosomiasis control in Zanzibar. The goals of the project are as follows: (1) to master the epidemiology of schistosomiasis in Pemba island and explore the localized comprehensive prevention methods and strategies of schistosomiasis control; (2) to eliminate the schistosomiasis as a public problem in project areas (Prevalence < 1%) by conducting effective schistosomiasis control activities; and (3) with the construction of practical and effective integrated of schistosomiasis control strategies, cooperate with Zanzibar and WHO to make a standard operating procedures (SOPs) for schistosomiasis control in Zanzibar.

From February 2017 to February 2020, 30 Chinese experts involved in the project of schistosomiasis control. To achieve these goals, the project helped local NTD office to scale up its ability of schistosomiasis control. The projected had renovated a new project office and laboratory which were equipped with advanced office and laboratory equipment. The office consisted of work rooms, rest rooms, and meeting rooms, it was equipped with new office supplies like computers, printers, projector, etc. Testing room and vector room are the major part of laboratory, which was equipped with microscopes, refrigerators, sample storage cabinets, centrifuges, dissecting microscopes, computers, etc. With the new office and laboratory, it provided a good base for carrying out schistosomiasis control activities. Some successful experience and methods like Geographic Information System (GIS) technology and computer-based schistosomiasis information system were trained to local team to scale up their abilities. By carrying out a comprehensive strategy including schistosomiasis infection source control and snail control and health promotion. The prevalence of schistosomiasis in all three project areas had reached the goal in 2 years, and the status can be maintained for a least 1 year. Patients were treated by watching them taking the medicine to secure the effect of treatment. By using new type of niclosamide and spraying machine, the infested snails were eliminated to zero in risk areas. Sound alarms and schistosomiasis control slogans were set up near communities and schools, and various types of health promotion and implementation activities had been carried out in cooperation with other departments. By implementing the schistosomiasis control water supply project, the project helped about 2500 people to get safe tap water, which also could help to control other kind of disease.

The project was evaluated by an international no-stakeholder expert group in May 2019. By reviewing data, listening to reports, field and laboratory visits, visiting schools and communities, and interviewing local government officials and the public, the project implementation plan, intermediate host control, team capacity building, population health education, data and information management, health economics, and other aspects were evaluated.

The evaluation team believed that the impact of interventions, reducing prevalence of infection below 1% in the intervention shehias over the 2-year period of the project, is the best that has ever been achieved in the island, and the work carried out during this pilot project has contributed to the establishment of WHO guidelines for laboratory and field testing of molluscicides for the control of schistosomiasis. They also thought that the success of the tripartite cooperation project will serve as a model for other African countries to learn from. This evaluation was also reported to the President of Zanzibar, Dr. Ali Mohamed Shein, who praised the contribution of the Chinese expert group, and said that he would continue to support Chinese experts and strive for the sustainable development of the project.

References

1. Zhou X-N. Tropical diseases in China schistosomiasis. Beijing, China: People's Medical Publishing House; 2018. ISBN: 978-7-117-25999-6.
2. Schistosomiasis in the People's Republic of China: from control to elimination.
3. Adenowo AF, Oyinloye BE, Ogunyinka BI, et al. Impact of human schistosomiasis in sub-Saharan Africa. Braz J Infect Dis. 2015;19(2):196–205.
4. Tzanetou K, Astriti M, Delis V, Moustakas G, et al. Intestinal schistosomiasis caused by both Schistosoma intercalatum and Schistosoma mansoni. Travel Med Infect Dis. 2010;8(3):184–9.
5. Lo NC, Addiss DG, Hotez PJ, et al. A call to strengthen the global strategy for schistosomiasis and soil-transmitted helminthiasis: the time is now. Lancet Infect Dis. 2017;17(2):e64–9. https://doi.org/10.1016/S1473-3099(16)30535-7.
6. Colley DG, Bustinduy AL, Secor WE, et al. Human schistosomiasis. Lancet. 2014;383:2253–64.
7. Schistosomiasis. Progress report 2001–2011 and strategic plan 2012–2020. Geneva: World Health Organization; 2013.
8. Simonsen PE, Fischer PU, Hoerauf A, et al. Manson's tropical diseases, 23rd Edition. Amsterdam: Elsevier; 2014. p. 698–725.
9. Steinmann P, Keiser J, Bos R, et al. Schistosomiasis and water resources development: systematic review, meta-analysis, and estimates of people at risk. Lancet Infect Dis. 2006;6:411–25.
10. World Health Organisation (WHO). PCT databank Schistosomiasis 2019. https://www.who.int/neglected_diseases/preventive_chemotherapy/sch/en. Accessed 18 Jan 2020.
11. Oyeyemi OT. Schistosomiasis control in Nigeria: moving round the circle? Ann Global Health. 2020;86(1):74, 1–3. https://doi.org/10.5334/aogh.2930.
12. Hotez PJ, Kamath A. Neglected tropical diseases in Sub-Saharan Africa: review of their prevalence, distribution, and disease burden. PLOS NTD. 2009;3(8):1–9.
13. Ezeh CO, Onyekwelu KC, et al. Urinary schistosomiasis in Nigeria: a 50 year review of prevalence, distribution and disease burden. Parasite. 2019;26:19.
14. Rollinsona D, Knopp S, Levitz S, et al. Time to set the agenda for schistosomiasis elimination. Acta Tropica. 2013;128:423–40.
15. Cunningham LJ, Campbell SJ, Armoo S, et al. Assessing expanded community wide treatment for schistosomiasis: baseline infection status and self-reported risk factors in three communities from the Greater Accra region, Ghana. PLOS NTD. 2020; https://doi.org/10.1371/journal.pntd.0007973.
16. Armoo S, Cunningham LJ, Campbell SJ, et al. Detecting Schistosoma mansoni infections among pre-school-aged children in southern Ghana: a diagnostic comparison of urine-CCA, real-time PCR and Kato-Katz assays. Infect Dis. 2020;20(301):1–10.

17. World Health Organisation (WHO). PCT bank Schistosomiasis 2018, https://www.who.int/neglected_diseases/preventive_chemotherapy/sch/en/.
18. WHO Western Pacific Region. Regional action framework for control and elimination of neglected tropical diseases in the Western Pacific. 2020. ISBN: 978 92 9061 907 9.
19. WHO. First WHO report on neglected tropical diseases 2010: working to overcome the global impact of neglected tropical diseases. Geneva: World Health Organization; 2010.
20. Adenowo AF, Oyinloye BE, Ogunyinka BI, et al. Impact of human schistosomiasis in sub-Saharan Africa. Braz J Infect Dis. 2015;19(2):196–205.
21. Mahmoud AAF. Schistosomiasis. Tropical medicine: science and practice. London: Imperial College Press; 2001.
22. Kosinski KC, Kulinkina AV, Tybor D, et al. Agreement among four prevalence metrics for urogenital schistosomiasis in the eastern region of Ghana. BioMed Res Int. 2016;7627358:1–11.
23. Wang W, Liang Y-S, Hong Q-B, et al. African schistosomiasis in mainland China: risk of transmission and countermeasures to tackle the risk. Parasit Vect. 2013;6:249.
24. Steiner F, Ignatius R, Friedrich-Jaenicke B, et al. Acute schistosomiasis in European students returning from fieldwork at Lake Tanganyika, Tanzania. J Travel Med. 2013;20(6):380–3. https://doi.org/10.1111/jtm.12069.
25. World Health Organization. Preventive chemotherapy in human helminthiasis. 2006.
26. World Health Organization. Field use of molluscicides in schistosomiasis control programmes.
27. Montresor A, Gabrielli AF, Chitsulo L, et al. Preventive chemotherapy and the fight against neglected tropical diseases. Exp Rev Anti-Infect Therapy. 10(2):237–42. https://doi.org/10.1586/eri.11.165.
28. Zhang Li-juan X, Zhi-Min DH, et al. Endemic status of schistosomiasis in People's Republic of China in 2019. Chin J Schist Control. 2020;32(6):551–8.
29. Mohamud A. Verjee. Schistosomiasis: still a cause of significant morbidity and mortality. Res Rep Trop Med. 2019;10:153–63.
30. Utzinger J, Bergquist R, Shu-Hua X, et al. Sustainable schistosomiasis control—the way forward. Lancet. 2003;362:1932–4.
31. Tchuenté L-AT, Rollinson D, Stothard JR, et al. Moving from control to elimination of schistosomiasis in sub-Saharan Africa: time to change and adapt strategies. Infect Dis Poverty. 2017;6:42.

COVID-19 Risk and Control 13

Jiandong Zheng and Luzhao Feng

Coronavirus disease 2019 (COVID-19) is a respiratory infection caused by the virus SARS-CoV-2. Coronaviruses (CoVs), enveloped positive-sense RNA viruses, are further subdivided into four different genera, historically based on serological analysis and now on genetic studies: alpha-, beta-, gamma-, and delta-CoV. The first two mainly infect mammals, while the second two mainly infect birds. There are currently seven known CoVs that can infect humans: HCoV-229E, HCoV-NL63, HCoV-OC43, HCoV-HKU1, SARS-CoV, MERS-CoV, and SARS-Cov-2. The last three are beta-CoVs, which are relatively high in infectivity and disease severity and pose a great threat to public health security in all countries. Current studies have shown that SARS-Cov-2 has already mutated into two lineages called "L-type" and "S-type." The phylogenetic tree indicates that the S-type is older than the L-type and more closely resembles bat coronaviruses. However, the L-type accounts for a larger proportion in the samples currently collected, suggesting that the recently evolved L-type spreads or replicates faster in human populations [1].

The clinical manifestations of COVID-19 patients are mainly respiratory symptoms, fever, chills, fatigue, diarrhea, conjunctival congestion, etc. Breathing difficulties and/or hypoxemia can occur in severe cases 1 week later, and critical patients rapidly progress to acute respiratory distress syndrome, sepsis, shock, metabolic acidosis, coagulation dysfunction, and multiple organ failure. Chest radiologic characteristics include multiple small patchy shadows and interstitial changes in the early stage, and then, multiple ground-glass opacity and patchy infiltrates in both lungs. Lung consolidation may appear in more severe cases, where pleural effusion is rare

J. Zheng
Chinese Center for Disease Control and Prevention, Beijing, People's Republic of China

L. Feng (✉)
Chinese Academy of Medical Sciences & Peking Union Medical College, Beijing, People's Republic of China
e-mail: fengluzhao@cams.cn

W. Yang (ed.), *Prevention and Control of Infectious Diseases in BRI Countries*,
https://doi.org/10.1007/978-981-33-6958-0_13

[2]. The main infection source of COVID-19 is patients and occasionally seen in the asymptomatic. SARS-Cov-2 mainly spreads through respiratory droplet and contact, or possibly, through aerosol when one is exposed to aerosols of high concentrations and for a long time in a relatively closed environment [2]. As a new infectious disease, people are generally susceptible to COVID-19 due to the lack of immunity, and we are still in the pandemic period. According to current epidemiological investigations and related research results, the latent period of COVID-19 is usually 1–14 days, and mostly 3–7 days. The basic regeneration index (R_0) is from 2 to 4.7. Its infectivity is strong on the onset, and also have infectivity at the end of the latent period [3]. Most of the deaths are patients aged 60 and above and suffer from underlying diseases, such as hypertension, cardiovascular disease, and diabetes [4].

The World Health Organization (WHO) announced COVID-19 a global pandemic on March 11, 2020. As of September 12, 2020, COVID-19 has spread to 216 countries and regions, with more than 28.2 million confirmed cases and over 900,000 deaths. Compared with SARS-CoV and MERS-CoV, although SARS-Cov-2 features milder clinical manifestations and lower case-fatality rate, it spreads much faster [5], hence the constant rise in the number of COVID-19 infections and deaths. COVID-19 has become the most widespread and severe global pandemic since the H1N1 influenza pandemic in 1918. It has not only brought a huge burden to medical and health systems worldwide, but also caused a huge impact on global economic development.

13.1 Overview of COVID-19 Pandemic in "Belt and Road" Countries

COVID-19 represents a global health crisis, and the pandemic is still spreading rapidly. Asia is the region first hit by the pandemic. In December 2019, when multiple cases of unexplained pneumonia were discovered in Wuhan, Hubei Province, China, the country immediately activated its joint prevention and control mechanism, adopted grid management policies, and implemented comprehensive prevention and control measures to block the spread of the epidemic in China. On March 2, 2020, the European Center for Disease Control and Prevention raised the risk level of COVID-19 to "high." WHO stated that Europe had become the "epicenter" of the COVID-19 pandemic. The total confirmed and dead cases reported by Europe exceeded the total of other countries and regions outside of China, and the number of cases reported daily was higher than that when the epidemic peaked in China. Although the spread of SARS-Cov-2 in Europe has slowed down after some time, the global pandemic is still on the rise and the situation is severe (see Fig. 13.1 [6]). The Americas, represented by the United States, followed Europe and became a new epicenter. As of September 12, 2020, the number of confirmed cases in the Americas and Brazil had exceeded 14.44 million, or 51.52% of the global total (14447680/28040853), becoming the continent with the largest number of confirmed cases and deaths. Among the "Belt and Road" countries, India has seen the largest number of confirmed cases of COVID-19 and is most affected by the epidemic, with over 4.56 million confirmed cases and nearly 90,000 new cases in a

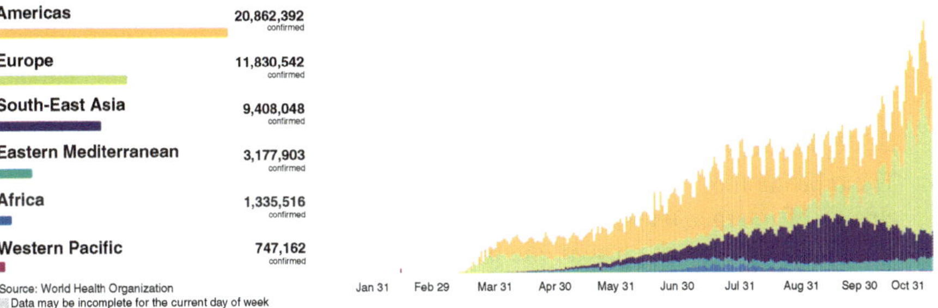

Fig. 13.1 Number of confirmed COVID-19 cases from January 1, 2020 to October 1, 2020 (by region). (Confirmed cases (10,000); Date; America; Southeast Asia)

single day. Its overall confirmed cases have exceeded Brazil and ranks second in the world. Other "Belt and Road" countries severely affected by the epidemic are Russia, Bangladesh, Saudi Arabia, Pakistan, Kazakhstan, and Iran. In the next 1–2 years, COVID-19 will maintain a high prevalence globally and a trend declining somewhere but possibly rising somewhere else. Facing economic globalization and integration, all countries and regions in the world must be prepared and ready to jointly prevent and control the spread of COVID-19.

13.2 COVID-19 Risk and Principles of Prevention and Control

13.2.1 Pandemic Risk

1. The transmission features of SARS-CoV-2 make some of its sources of infection relatively "hidden" and difficult for timely detection. Moreover, there is a risk of clusters of cases and even community transmission caused by local residual sources of infection and imported infections from abroad. SARS-CoV-2 is highly contagious, peaking 2 days before the onset to 1 week after the onset. Patients may feel in the early stage that the symptoms are mild and do not need to go to see a doctor. Besides, the untypical symptoms of the infected person and the difficulty in timely discovery of the source of infection make it possible in reality that transmission starts before the case is discovered and managed in isolation.
2. The sensitivity of the surveillance system of healthcare institutions needs to be improved. If all types of medical institutions, especially key "sentinel" departments of primary medical institutions such as fever clinics, respiratory medicine department, and emergency departments, fail to execute in an effective manner the first-diagnosis responsibility system, or the time taken for the investigation of suspected patients from sample collection to laboratory diagnosis is too long, the patients may not be properly administered, which may in turn cause familial cluster, nosocomial infection, or even spread to the community.
3. Medical institutions at all levels are faced with different degrees of nosocomial infection risks. The spread in medical institutions can be easy due to the rela-

tively closed environment, the heavy flow of people, and the large number of susceptible populations. In addition, without basic nosocomial protection and screening measures for suspected infections, SARS-CoV-2 infected patients with other diseases and treated or hospitalized in non-infectious departments may bring great risks of nosocomial infection.

4. The relaxation of measures and public awareness of protection can increase the chance of interpersonal contact, hence rising risks of infection. In view of the low epidemic level at present, the public may relax their vigilance, neglect the use of personal preventive measures, or gather together more with others, which all will increase the chance of infection and transmission.
5. As disease control and prevention agencies at all levels are understaffed, without adequate professionals for emergencies over a long term, the pandemic response is low in speed and efficiency. Community prevention and control also face similar problems.
6. COVID-19 as a pandemic is still in its early stages, and will remain severe for at least 2 years. Without specific medicine, the immune barrier of people is established in two ways: natural infection or vaccination. Given the uncertainty of the latter, even if vaccines can be developed soon, there are still potential safety, effectiveness, and productivity issues, while an immune barrier formed through natural infection will require a huge price and quite long [7].

13.2.2 Principles of Prevention and Control

13.2.2.1 General Requirements and Principles

In the early stage of the pandemic, community mobilization, adopt grid-based, carpet-style management, and observe the "4 Earlies," that is, early detection, early reporting, and early isolation/quarantine for early diagnosis and treatment were given to fully played [8]. In the normalized prevention and control stage, the overall prevention and control strategy of "preventing importation of cases, avoiding a resurgence of local cases," and timely detection, rapid disposal, targeted control, and effective treatment were implemented [9].

13.2.2.2 Specific Requirements and Principles

13.2.2.2.1 Put Prevention in the First Place

1. Wear masks properly. Wear a mask when you are in close contact with others within a distance of less than 1 m in crowded closed places.
2. Reduce gatherings. Keep a social distance of more than 1 m. Reduce unnecessary gatherings and the number of people in gatherings. Try not to go to places and especially closed places where people gather.
3. Increase ventilation and disinfection. Frequently open windows for ventilation in the room to maintain air circulation. Hygienic measures such as daily cleaning and disinfection must be implemented in public places, stations, docks, and public transportation.

4. Improve health etiquette. Develop hygiene habits and lifestyles such as keeping "one-meter socializing distance," washing hands frequently, wearing masks, and using serving chopsticks. Cover the nose and mouth with tissues or the elbow when coughing or sneezing.

13.2.2.2.2 Implement the "4 Earlies" Measures

1. Early detection. Measure body temperature in public places, strengthen pre-screening, triage and fever clinic investigations for "early detection" of confirmed cases, suspected cases, asymptomatic infections, and then "early report" as required. No late, left-out or concealed reports are allowed.
2. Quick disposal. Complete the epidemiological investigation within 24 h, tap the advantages of big data, etc., so as to identify possible sources of infection as soon as possible, discover and track close contacts. Implement "early isolation" measures to timely isolate and treat confirmed and suspected cases, and for asymptomatic infections and close contacts, implement centralized medical observation for 14 days. Carry out thorough disinfection of possible contaminated places.
3. Targeted control. Scientifically delineate the prevention and control area to the smallest unit (building, ward, residential area, natural village, etc.), and decisively adopt measures such as restricting gatherings of people, blockade, and cut off the route of transmission to minimize the risk of infection. Promptly announce relevant information of the prevention and control area.
4. Effective treatment. Designate hospitals for admission and treatment, implement "early treatment" measures. Admit and treat mild cases in a timely and effective manner, reduce their conversion to severe ones. Adhere to the "4 Concentrations," provide multidisciplinary treatment to severe cases. Maximize the cure rate and reduce the mortality rate. After the patient is cured and discharged from the hospital, implement 14-day medical observation in home quarantine or a concentrated manner.

13.2.2.2.3 Highlight Key Links

1. Prevention and control at key places. In accordance with relevant technical guidelines, and under the premise of implementing prevention and control measures, fully open shopping malls, supermarkets, hotels, restaurants, and other living places. Adopt appointments and flow restriction measures when opening parks, tourist attractions, sports venues, indoor venues such as libraries, museums, art galleries, and closed entertainment and leisure venues, such as theaters and amusement halls. All kinds of necessary meetings, exhibitions, etc., can be held.
2. Prevention and control of key institutions. Prevent risks in nursing institutions for the aged, welfare homes, prisons, mental healthcare institutions, and implement prevention and control measures such as entry and exit management, personnel protection, health monitoring, and disinfection.
3. Prevention and control of key population groups. Instruct key groups such as the elderly, children, pregnant women, the disabled, and patients with severe chronic

diseases in personal protection, and offer psychological counseling, care, and assistance.

4. Medical institution prevention and control. Strengthen the prevention and control of nosocomial infections, promote time-phased appointments for diagnosis and treatment, strictly implement community management requirements for medical institutions, promptly investigate risks and take measures. Strictly manage visits and escorts to avoid cross-infection. Be strict with prescreening, triage, and fever clinic work processes, implement protective measures for healthcare workers, and strengthen health management and monitoring of them.
5. School prevention and control. Implement a "daily report" and "zero report" mechanism for the health of faculty, staff, and students. Provide health tips, carry out health management, classroom ventilation, disinfection, etc., and measure body temperatures of kindergartners and students in the morning and at noon. Track and register cause of illness of those absent from school (duty).
6. Community prevention and control. Strengthen the grid management of grassroots communities and tap the role of community volunteers. Offer health education and manage environmental sanitation, rented houses, dormitories, and non-native population. Communities where the outbreak has occurred should strengthen the investigation, isolation, and terminal disinfection of close contacts, and take such measures as restricting gatherings of people and closed management when necessary.

13.2.2.2.4 Strengthen Support

1. Expand the scope of detection. Make scientific assessments based on detection capabilities and as needed in prevention and control. Detect key populations such as close contacts, overseas immigrants, fever clinic patients, newly hospitalized patients and accompanying persons, medical institution staff, port quarantine and border inspection personnel, etc., that should be detected. For other people, detect "whoever want to."
2. Employ big data. Rely on information service platforms for timely sharing of nucleic acid and serum antibody test results and data on key personnel to the electronic database. Promote the safe and orderly flow of personnel. Promote and apply the version for people entering China, and carry out closed-loop management of them.
3. Strengthen scientific research and international cooperation. Promote research on vaccines, pharmaceutical science and technology, virus mutation, and immune strategies. Speed up the development of detection reagents and equipment, improve sensitivity, specificity, and simplicity. Further enhance detection capabilities and shorten detection time. Strengthen information sharing, technical exchanges, and prevention and control cooperation with international organizations like WHO and relevant countries.

13.2.2.2.5 Strengthen Organization and Leadership

1. Allocate responsibilities to institutions and units. Implement territorial responsibilities, strengthen organization and leadership, increase funding, strengthen the

dynamic reserve of medical supplies, and improve capacities in prevention, control, and emergency response.

2. Dynamic adjustment of the level of risk and emergency response. All localities shall dynamically adjust the level of risk and emergency response according to classification standards and local transmission situation. Adapt measures to local conditions and circumstances, and constantly improve the prevention and control emergency plan and various supporting work plans. Once there is an outbreak, emergency response measures shall be taken in time, followed by targeted prevention and control [9].

13.3 Case Study

China's Response to the First Wave of COVID-19 Epidemic

1. Overview

Four pandemics have appeared in the world since the twentieth century, and the most serious one was the Spanish pandemic in 1918, causing approximately 20–50 million deaths worldwide [10]. The COVID-19 epidemic is a major public health emergency. The virus has spread faster and wider than any other since the founding of the People's Republic in 1949, and has proven to be the most difficult to contain. It is both a crisis and a major test for China. Under the leadership of the Communist Party of China, the whole nation has followed the general principle of "remaining confident, coming together in solidarity, adopting a science-based approach, and taking targeted measures," and waged an all-out people's war on the virus. Through painstaking efforts and tremendous sacrifice, and having paid a heavy price, China has succeeded in turning the situation around. In little more than a single month, the rising spread of the virus was contained; in around 2 months, the daily increase in domestic coronavirus cases had fallen to single digits; and in approximately 3 months, a decisive victory was secured in the battle to defend Hubei Province and its capital city of Wuhan. With these strategic achievements, China has protected its people's lives, safety and health, and made a significant contribution to safeguarding regional and global public health.

2. Prevention and Control Stages and Strategic Measures [11]

The prevention and control of COVID-19 in China can be roughly divided into five stages:

Stage 1, swift response to the Public Health Emergency (December 27, 2019 to January 19, 2020). When cases of pneumonia of unknown cause were monitored in Wuhan City, Hubei Province, China reported the epidemic the first time, and promptly took scientific and epidemiological investigations to stop the spread of the disease. It spared no time in reporting the epidemic to WHO, the United States, and other countries, and announced the sequence of the virus to the world. As localized community transmission and clusters of cases occurred in Wuhan, and Wuhan-associated confirmed cases began to appear in other areas, China embarked on thorough epidemic prevention and control.

Stage 2, initial progress in containing the virus (January 20 to February 20). The number of new confirmed cases nationwide increased rapidly, and the prevention and control situation got extremely severe. China took a key move to stop the spread of the virus by resolutely closing passage from Wuhan and Hubei, commencing the war to defend Wuhan and Hubei. The Central Committee of the Communist Party set up a leading group for response to the epidemic and deployed a central steering group to Hubei and other severely affected areas. The State Council successively established a joint prevention and control mechanism and a working mechanism for resuming work and production. The whole country gathered its resources and strength and rushed to assist Hubei and Wuhan. Localities initiated emergency response to major public health emergencies. The most comprehensive, rigorous, and thorough national epidemic prevention and control was officially launched, and the spread of the epidemic was initially contained.

Stage 3, newly confirmed domestic cases on the Chinese mainland drop to single digits (February 21 to March 17). At this stage, the rapid spread of the virus had been contained in Wuhan and the rest of Hubei Province, the situation in other parts on the mainland had stabilized, and the daily figure for new cases had remained in single digits since mid-March. As the situation evolved, the Central Committee made a major decision to coordinate epidemic prevention and control, economic and social development, and orderly resume work and production.

Stage 4, Wuhan and Hubei—an initial victory in a critical battle (March 18 to April 28). The spread of the national epidemic with Wuhan as the main battlefield was basically blocked, and the control measures for the passage from Wuhan and Hubei were lifted. Wuhan cleared the number of COVID-19 patients in the hospital, and the defense war of Wuhan and Hubei achieved decisive results, and major strategic results of the country in epidemic prevention and control. The epidemic spread sporadically at home, but rapidly overseas. Imported cases from abroad caused the spread of related cases. On this situation, the Central Committee determined the prevention and control strategy of "preventing importation of cases, avoiding a resurgence of local cases," consolidated and furthered the effectiveness of domestic epidemic prevention and control, timely dealt with clusters of epidemics, promoted the resumption of work and production by categories, and cared for overseas Chinese citizens in need.

Stage 5, ongoing prevention and control (April 29 to present). Sporadic cases have been reported on the mainland, resulting in case clusters in some locations. Imported cases from abroad are basically under control, and the epidemic situation continues to be active. The national epidemic prevention and control has become normalized. Further efforts are made to promote the resumption of work, production, and schooling.

3. Experiences

Since the beginning of COVID-19 outbreak, China has adopted two response strategies—containment and suppression, both of which have adopted considerable non-pharmaceutical interventions [3]. It has fully tapped the capacities of community mobilization, implement grid-based, carpet-style management, all-people prevention and control, stable and targeted prevention and control, and comprehensive measures for "early detection, early reporting, early investigation, early isolation, early diagnosis, and early treatment" to prevent the import, spread, and export of the epidemic, and control its spread.

Five pieces of main experiences:

One, take firm and effective measures to control the source of infection and reduce the infection rate. Revise six versions of COVID-19 prevention and control plans. Adopt strict isolation and control measures for four categories of people—confirmed cases, suspected cases, fever patients, and close contacts—so as to admit, test, treat, and isolate whoever in need. The practice has proved that detecting and isolating cases, tracing and isolating close contacts for medical observation have been the most effective measures of containment strategy, when comparing with travel restrictions and contact reduction, and can prevent more people from infection. These measures can work even better when combined with other non-pharmaceutical interventions, such as reducing the movement of people (traffic control and travel restrictions, etc.), keep social distancing (stopping large-scale activities, delaying the opening of schools and the resumption of work in factories), and encouraging personal prevention [12].

Two, speed up testing. Devolve the authority to detect infectious diseases from CDC testing to all Level 2 and above hospitals, increase laboratories, cultivate personnel, and at the same time, use third parties to strengthen the testing work. Form a closed-loop system to "complete network report in 2 h, detection information feedback in 12 h, and epidemiological survey in 24 h." At the beginning of the epidemic, the average interval between the diagnosis of a patient was 15.4 days, and in mid-term, 3 days, hence the sharp decline in the probability of disease transmission. The epidemiological survey and closed-loop system have enabled us to grasp the initiative in the control of the epidemic.

Three, manage to ensure the supply of medical services and increase the admission rate. Designate over 2000 medical institutions and intensive care hospitals nationwide, and more than 10,000 fever clinics. Increase hospital beds in Wuhan and establish an emergency treatment network with a tiered layout of designated hospitals, mobile hospitals, and isolation points. Build Huoshenshan and Leishenshan hospitals, and transform general hospitals such as Tongji Hospital, Union Hospital, and Hubei Provincial People's Hospital. Mobile hospitals have played a very important role in admitting mild cases, so that patients found out in community screening could be admitted to the hospital. With three main features (rapid in construction, large in scale, low in cost) and five basic functions (isolation, classification, basic medical care, frequent monitoring and quick referral, and basic life and social participation) [13], they admitted whoever in need in the epidemic [11]. The disaster prevention hospital they represent is an important part of the national response to the COVID-19 pandemic, and such a role may continue in future epidemics and public health emergencies [13].

Four, add isolation points. Transform more than 630 hotels, schools, training centers, and medical institutions into isolation rooms for close contacts and suspected patients, take effective isolation measures, and implement prevention and control measures.

Five, go all out to treat patients, increase the cure rate, and reduce the mortality rate. China has carried out large-scale medical rescue work, with 346 national medical teams, 42,000 medical workers, and 19,000 critical care medical workers rushing to Hubei and Wuhan for assistance. The national team takes over all severe cases, restructure systems and takes over ICUs, with doctors from the Department of Intensive Medicine, Respiratory Medicine, Circulatory Medicine and Infection Department serving as the main force. The treatment of severe cases in a concentrated manner has been constantly improved, and traditional Chinese and western medicine are combined in mobile hospitals to treat mild cases and prevent them from becoming severe ones.

Implement "Five Combinations." First, combine basic medicine and clinical medicine. Second, combine the front and the rear. In case of problems with the medical work in the front, a video connection is made from the rear, and multi-disciplinary support is provided to mobilize key disciplines across the country to support Wuhan. Third, combine doctors and nurses. Fourth, combine medical treatment and management, which is also a major feature in the epidemic, when more than 42,000 medical staff with strong expertise, professionalism and administrative command ability, worked in the epidemic area in an orderly manner. Fifth, vertical administrative leadership system. Establish medical department, nursing department, and hospital control department. None of the 42,000 medical staff were infected. And the mobile hospital has realized zero deaths, zero infections, and zero recurrences. Traditional Chinese medicine has played a significant role, and the medical workers dared the disease and shown the spirit of self-sacrifice.

Thanks to the above prevention and treatment measures, China has significantly reduced the incidence and mortality of COVID-19, and successfully contained the continuous spread of COVID-19 virus in the community. Given the extremely low infection rate in China, currently, the vast majority of people are still vulnerable to COVID-19 infection. Therefore, it is necessary to carry forward public health measures to prevent infections. Meantime, China is developing vaccines and specific therapeutic drugs, and adopting prevention and control measures that have the least impact on social production and life. These experiences have consolidated the country's confidence in defeating the epidemic and are conducive to containing the next wave of the COVID-19 epidemic [14].

References

1. Tang X, Wu C, Li X, et al. On the origin and continuing evolution of SARS-CoV-2. Natl Sci Rev. 2020;6(7):1012–23. https://doi.org/10.1093/nsr/nwaa036.
2. The National Health Commission of the People's Republic of China. Notice on issuing COVID-19 diagnosis and treatment plan (trial version 7). [EB/OL] [2020-07-10] http://www.nhc.gov.cn/yzygj/s7653p/202003/46c9294a7dfe4cef80dc7f5912eb1989.shtml.
3. Li Z, Chen Q, Feng L, et al. Active case finding with case management: the key to tackling the COVID-19 pandemic.[J]. Lancet. 2020;396(10243):63–70. https://doi.org/10.1016/S0140-6736(20)31278-2.
4. Epidemiology Group of COVID-19 Emergency Response Mechanism, China CDC. Analysis of epidemiological characteristics of COVID-19 [J]. Chin J Epidemiol. 2020;41(2):145–51. https://doi.org/10.3760/cma.j.issn.0254-6450.2020.02.003.
5. Zhu B, Feng P, Li F, et al. Research progress of the etiology and clinical epidemiology of three newly discovered coronaviruses [J/OL]. Chin J Nosocomiol. 2020;15:2274–80. [2020-07-09]. http://kns.cnki.net/kcms/detail/11.3456.R.20200702.0906.016.html.
6. World Health Organization. Coronavirus disease (COVID-19) Situation Report—162 [EB/OL] [2020-07-10]. https://www.who.int/docs/default-source/coronaviruse/20200630-covid-19-sitrep-162.pdf?sfvrsn=e00a5466_2.
7. World Health Organization. Coronavirus disease (COVID-19) Situation Report—163 2020; [EB/OL] [2020-07-10]. https://www.who.int/docs/default-source/coronaviruse/situation-reports/20200701-covid-19-sitrep-163.pdf?sfvrsn=c202f05b_2.
8. The National Health Commission. Notice on strengthening community prevention and control of COVID-19 epidemic. [EB/OL] [2020-07-10] 2020. http://www.nhc.gov.cn/jkj/s3577/202001/dd1e502534004a8d88b6a10f329a3369.shtml.
9. The State Council's Joint Prevention and Control Mechanism for COVID-19 Epidemic. Guiding opinions of the State Council on the normalization of COVID-19 epidemic prevention and control. [EB/OL] [2020-07-10]. http://www.gov.cn/gongbao/content/2020/content_5512557.htm?luicode=10000011&lfid=1076032927573465&u=http%3A%2F%2Fwww.gov.cn%2Fgongbao%2Fcontent%2F2020%2Fcontent_5512557.htm.
10. Qin Y, Zhao M, Tan Y, et al. Influenza pandemic over a hundred year in China [J]. Chin J Epidemiol. 2018;39(08):1028–31. https://doi.org/10.3760/cma.j.issn.0254-6450.2018.08.003.
11. The Information Office of the State Council of the People's Republic of China. China action against COVID-19 epidemic. [EB/OL] [2020-07-10]. http://www.scio.gov.cn/ztk/dtzt/42313/43142/index.htm.
12. Chen W, Wang Q, Li Y, et al. Overview of early containment strategies for COVID-19 epidemic in China [J]. Chin J Prevent Med. 2020;3:239–44. https://doi.org/10.3760/cma.j.issn.0253-9624.2020.03.003.
13. Chen S, Zhang Z, Yang J, et al. Fangcang shelter hospitals: a novel concept for responding to public health emergencies. Lancet. 2020;395(10232):1305–14. https://doi.org/10.1016/S0140-6736(20)30744-3.
14. Zhou L, Wu Z, Li Z, et al. 100 Days of COVID-19 prevention and control in China. Clin Infect Dis. 2020;2020:ciaa725. https://doi.org/10.1093/cid/ciaa725.

14 Risk of AIDS and Its Prevention and Control

Guang Zhang and Weizhong Yang

AIDS, or acquired immunodeficiency syndrome, is a malignant infectious disease caused by human immunodeficiency virus (HIV) with a very high mortality rate. Once HIV enters the body, it can destroy the body's immune system. HIV attacks the CD4+T lymphocytes (CD4 cells), which are critical to the immune system, leaving the body vulnerable to life-threatening infections and cancers. The mean incubation period of HIV is 8–10 years. When HIV remains dormant, people with it can live and work for many years without any symptoms of the infection. There is no vaccine yet developed for HIV infection, and there is no cure. HIV, the virus that causes AIDS, remains one of the most serious health challenges worldwide [1].

HIV, which can survive in body fluids and attack the body's immune system, is a single-stranded, enveloped RNA retrovirus. HIV is currently divided into two types, HIV-1 and HIV-2, according to the genetic diversity [2]. HIV-1 is widely disseminated worldwide and plays a major role in the global AIDS epidemic, while HIV-2 is concentrated in Africa, but has been seen in Europe, North America, South America, India, and some countries in Asia. Between the two types of HIV, HIV-1 is more reproducible, has a higher rate of transmission, and causes more severe clinical symptoms. HIV-1 is further classified into four groups (M, N, O and P). M is the "major" group and is responsible for the majority of the global HIV epidemic. Within

The original version of this chapter was revised. A correction to this chapter is available at https://doi.org/10.1007/978-981-33-6958-0_15

G. Zhang
National Center for AIDS/STD Control and Prevention, China CDC, Beijing, People's Republic of China

W. Yang (✉)
Chinese Academy of Medical Sciences & Peking Union Medical College, Chinese Preventive Medicine Association, The UN Consultative Committee on Life Science and Human Health (CCLH) of China Association of Science and Technology (CAST), Beijing, P.R China
e-mail: yangwz@chinacdc.cn

W. Yang (ed.), *Prevention and Control of Infectious Diseases in BRI Countries*, https://doi.org/10.1007/978-981-33-6958-0_14

group M, there are known to be at least 11 genetically distinct subtypes of HIV-1 (subtypes A-K) and different epidemic recombinant forms (CRFs). The other three groups—N, O and P—are mainly confined to Central Africa and have a low prevalence. HIV-2 has at least 7 subtypes, A–G. HIV subtypes are of great significance in the studies of the prevalence and distribution of AIDS, and its clinical treatment, diagnostic, drug screening, and vaccine development. In China, HIV-1 is the prevalent virus, HIV-1 subtypes CRF01_AE, CRF07_BC and B′ are predominant, and the subtype distribution varies in different regions. The prevalent strains in northwest and central China are relatively single, with CRF07_BC the most widely distributed in the northwest, and the B′ overwhelming in the central. Three subtypes are prevalent in northeast, north, east, and south China: CRF01_AE, CRF07_BC, and B′. The distribution of HIV-1 subtypes in southwest China is relatively complex, mainly CRF08_BC and CRF01_AE, followed by CRF07_BC, and other subtypes also account for a considerable proportion. From the perspective of people infected by different viral transmission routes, the HIV-1 subtypes of blood-borne infections are relatively unitary, mainly B′. Among the drug users, the dominant strain is CRF07_BC, CRF01_AE, and CRF08_BC subtypes which account for a certain proportion; among homosexual males, the predominant strain is CRF01_AE; among the heterosexually transmitted population, the distribution of prevalent HIV-1 strains is relatively complex, with all subtypes found. The relationship between the transmissibility of different subtypes of HIV-1 and disease progression is not clear.

The source of HIV infection consists of AIDS patients and HIV sufferers, and there is no evidence that other people or animals can transmit HIV. As a source of infection, people in different stages of HIV infection or disease progression have different viral transmission capacities due to different HIV viral loads in their plasma, and antiviral drugs also have a significant impact on the spread of HIV [3].

After 2–4 weeks of HIV infection, the infected person will have a high viral load, and some people may have some non-specific clinical symptoms and signs, such as fever, and the body has not yet fully produced HIV antibody. At this stage, the infected person, with relatively strong virus transmissibility, is the most dangerous source of infection. In recent years, it has been found that when human beings are infected with HIV, there is a period when HIV antibodies cannot be detected in the serum, which may be that the antibody concentration in the body is not enough or antibodies have not yet been produced. At this point, the correct results cannot be obtained, and it must take some time before HIV antibodies can be detected. But there is HIV in the body and it is infectious, and this is the so-called window period. According to the Diagnosis of AIDS and HIV Infection issued by China's Health Commission in 2019 [4], "the window period is from when a person is infected with HIV to when markers of infection such as HIV antibodies, antigens or nucleic acids in his/her serum can be detected." Blood is infectious during the window period, and the window period of detection of HIV antibodies, antigens, and nucleic acids by the available diagnostic techniques is about 3 weeks, 2 weeks, and 1 week after infection, respectively.

After the acute infection period, the human body produces antibodies to HIV, the viral load in the body drops to a relatively low level, and the body is in a relatively balanced state with HIV. At this time, the HIV-infected person has a relatively weak virus transmissibility. However, due to the long duration of this stage, which lasts for 10–20 years, the viral load in the body changes greatly and the infected person can live normally, but the risk of virus transmission remains high. When the human body enters the onset period, the viral load in the body is at a high level, at which time the virus transmissibility is strong, but due to the relatively weak mobility of the infected person as a source of disease infection, his/her virus transmissibility as a source of infection is correspondingly reduced. After effective treatment, the virus in HIV sufferers and AIDS patients can be controlled at a relatively low level. At this time, their virus transmissibility is relatively low. If treatment fails or drug resistance develops, the viral load will rise rapidly, and their virus transmissibility will increase, and it may cause the prevalence of drug-resistant HIV strains.

HIV is mainly found in blood, semen, vaginal secretions, tissue fluids, cerebrospinal fluid, lymph, breast milk, and other body fluids of the infected persons. It can be transmitted through three routes, including heterosexual and male–male transmission, iatrogenic transmission and blood infection (including intravenous infusion of HIV-contaminated blood, blood components, or blood products and intravenous drug use), and mother-to-child transmission. Although HIV has been isolated from saliva, tears, urine and sweat, such body fluids are not responsible for the spread of AIDS. There is no evidence that HIV can be transmitted through other routes than the above three.

People in populations who are at increased HIV risk are generally referred to as high-risk populations. The current definition of the populations who are at increased HIV risk in China's integrated surveillance system for AIDS and sexually transmitted diseases include female sex workers, drug users, men who have sex with men, STD patients, and paid blood donors [5].

14.1 HIV/AIDS Epidemic in the Countries of the Belt and Road Initiative

Studies suggest that HIV originated in Africa and was brought into the United States by immigrants. On June 5, 1981, an article published in the CDC's Morbidity and Mortality Weekly Report (MMWR) describes five cases of an unusual form of pneumonia that later became known as AIDS, which is the first official record of AIDS in the world. In 1982, the disease was named AIDS. Before long, AIDS spread rapidly to all continents through travelers. In 1985, a foreigner visiting China died soon after being admitted to Peking Union Medical College Hospital and was later confirmed to have died of AIDS, which was the first case of AIDS found in China. After 146 drug users in Ruili, a city in Dehong Prefecture, southwestern Yunnan Province on the edge of the "Golden Triangle" region of traditional drug trafficking, were found to be infected with HIV in 1989, HIV spread through several counties in Dehong Prefecture. At this stage, HIV infection among intravenous drug users was found in several areas such as Ruili, presenting a regional cluster and spreading mainly in border areas. After 1995, HIV prevalence among intravenous drug users appeared in Yunnan, Guangxi, Xinjiang, Sichuan and other provinces/regions, and rapidly expanded to most provinces (autonomous regions and municipalities directly under the Central Government). In the central provinces, HIV infection occurred mainly among people who with illegal blood supply, and spread to more areas through population movements and second-generation transmission. In developed coastal areas and large and medium-sized cities, HIV is mainly transmitted sexually.

In recent years, the HIV/AIDS epidemic in China has shown a trend of mainly through sexual transmission, and the proportion of blood transmission and intravenous drug use has significantly decreased. The overall level of HIV/AIDS epidemic is low. In 2018, a total of 861,042 persons living with HIV/AIDS were reported nationwide. It is estimated that 1.25 million people (1.1–1.4 million) are living with HIV/AIDS, with an infection rate in the whole population of about 0.09%. One of the features of HIV/AIDS epidemic in China is mainly through sexual transmission. In 2018, 94.8% of newly reported cases were sexually transmitted, with heterosexual transmission accounting for 71.5% and homosexual transmission among males accounting for 23.3%. The second feature is the large regional differences. By the end of 2018, there were 22 provinces with more than 10,000 persons living with HIV/AIDS. In 2018, there were nine provinces with the proportion of heterosexual transmission exceeding 70% of the newly reported cases and six provinces with the proportion of homosexual transmission exceeding 70%. The third feature is the number of infected males aged over 60 years on the rise. The number of infected men aged 60 and above increased from 4751 in 2010 to 24,465 in 2018, accounting for 16.5% of the total number of reported cases in 2018, up from 7.4% in 2010.

The distribution of HIV/AIDS varies across continents and the trends vary too, with sub-Saharan Africa still the region with the most severe HIV infection. In 2006, sub-Saharan Africa has nearly 25 million HIV-infected persons, accounting for 63% of those infected worldwide. Although the availability of antiviral drugs has greatly improved, 2.1 million HIV-infected people died of AIDS, accounting for 3/4 of the global AIDS deaths that year. This region as a whole has seen a steady increase in HIV infection rates in recent years, with more than 15% of adults infected in Botswana, Lesotho, Namibia, South Africa, Zimbabwe, and Swaziland. The number of children under the age of 15 infected with HIV worldwide increased from 1.6 million in 2001 to 2 million in 2007, with 90% living in sub-Saharan Africa. A new situation has emerged in some countries in sub-Saharan Africa where injecting drug use has become a potential risk factor for the HIV epidemic, particularly in South Africa. HIV prevalence in East Africa is much lower than in South Africa, and the overall epidemic tends to stabilize or decline. HIV prevalence among pregnant women has declined in Kenya, is similar in Tanzania and slightly lower in Rwanda. While in other countries, differences tend to show up in different parts of the country, with prevalence rising in rural areas of some countries. It is estimated that in 2019, 20.7 million people (18.4 million to 23 million) are living with HIV/

AIDS in east and south Africa, 730,000 people (580,000–940,000) were newly infected that year, and 300,000 (230,000–390,000) died of AIDS-related diseases. Although new HIV infections in this region have declined substantially since 2010, gender inequalities in HIV epidemic are still to be addressed. In 2019, 3/5 of the new infections were in women, and young women aged 15–24 had an unusually high rate of new infections than men. Besides comprehensive interventions, there is an urgent need to address the rise in new HIV infections among women through measures such as addressing gender inequality, sexual and reproductive health issues, and primary education.

The HIV epidemic is on the rise in Eastern Europe and Central Asia, where are currently among the fastest growing regions of HIV infection in the world. In 2007, there were 1.5 million HIV infections, a 36% increase over 2003, 110,000 new infections, and 58,000 AIDS-related deaths, more than double the number in 2003. This is mainly because the increase in the number of infected people in Ukraine and Russia is the most significant in the whole of Europe. The HIV epidemic in such countries mainly affects young people, and drug use with unsterilized syringes is the major pattern of HIV transmission. In Russia, 80% of those infected with HIV are young people under the age of 30, and the majority of women under 25 years of age in Ukraine and Russia are under serious threat of HIV infection, with an increasing rate of infection. In Central Asia, Tajikistan and Uzbekistan are with relatively mild outbreaks. In 2019, it is estimated that in the Eastern European and Central Asian countries, 1.7 million (1.4 million to 1.9 million) people are living with HIV, 170,000 (140,000–190,000) were newly infected that year, and 35,000 (26,000–45,000) died of AIDS-related diseases. Eastern Europe and Central Asia are among the only three regions where the AIDS epidemic is growing, and there is an urgent need to expand HIV prevention services, particularly in Russia, and there is a large gap between HIV testing and initiation of treatment. Only 63% (52–71%) of those living with HIV in this region who know they are living with HIV are receiving treatment, and only 41% (34–46%) of all HIV-infected people in this region have experienced viral suppression after receiving antiviral treatment. Significant efforts are needed to reverse current trends, including increased provision of community-based HIV intervention services focused on the most severely affected population, such as HIV self-testing, injury reduction and pre-exposure prophylaxis (PrEP).

Compared with other continents worldwide, Asia and the Pacific region have a lower HIV infection rate and a population-wide HIV prevalence of less than 1%, but with 60% of the world's population, Asia will have a huge impact on the global AIDS epidemic as a result of the growth of the epidemic in this region. In recent years, the increasing prevalence of AIDS in Central, South, and Southeast Asia has attracted global attention. In 2019, an estimated 5.8 million people (4.3–7.2 million) are living with HIV in Asia and the Pacific region, 300,000 (210,000–39,000) were newly infected that year, and 160,000 (94,000–240,000) died of AIDS-related diseases. Thailand, Cambodia, and Myanmar are among the countries in Asia where the HIV/AIDS epidemic began earlier, but the rate of increase of HIV infection in these countries has been declining in recent years, mainly due to continuous comprehensive HIV interventions, including promoting condom use, resisting and combating commercial sex, and conducting public health education. But HIV infections are rising fast in Indonesia, Pakistan, and Vietnam. The high-prevalence region in Asia is southeast Asia, where unprotected commercial sex, male–male sex, unsafe injecting drug use, and the interaction of several high-risk behaviors are the most risk factors for the AIDS epidemic. The prevalence of HIV among men who have sex with men (MSM) is increasing in Southeast Asia, such as in Cambodia, India, Nepal, Pakistan, Vietnam, and Thailand. Due to social, religious, and cultural reasons, only a few countries have made detailed investigations and taken targeted measures on the prevalence of HIV among MSM. The HIV outbreak in Afghanistan and Pakistan, particularly among injecting drug users, is the result of unsterilized syringes and other risky behaviors.

Over the past four decades, the epidemic situation and mode of transmission of HIV/AIDS have been constantly changing, and interventions to prevent HIV transmission have been constantly explored, promoted, and updated [6]. In particular, in the past 10 years, global HIV prevention has expanded from previous preventive interventions such as publicity and education, behavioral interventions, harm reduction measures, and condom promotion to the treatment of people living with HIV so that their viral load can be controlled at undetectable levels (Undetectable = Untran smittable, or U = U), and providing antiviral treatment to uninfected persons before and after high-risk behavior to prevent infection (PrEP and nPEP). In China, HIV transmission through blood transfusion has been basically blocked, and the number of HIV cases infected through blood transfusion is close to zero. The spread of HIV through injecting drug use has been effectively controlled, with the number of injecting drug users infected decreasing year by year (4426 cases), accounting for 3% of those infected through various transmission routes. The rate of new infections among patients with methadone maintenance treatment (MMT) has decreased to 0.03%. The transmission of HIV through mother-to-child has been effectively controlled, with a transmission rate dropped to 4.5%, the lowest level in history. However, sexually transmitted cases account for the vast majority of newly reported HIV infections, and there is still no sign of control and end of the epidemic. As the number of people tested in China increases year by year, so does the number of newly diagnosed HIV infections, and the intensity of testing is constantly increasing. In 2018, a total of 240 million HIV tests were conducted, and 149,000 new infections were detected [7]. For the promotion and application of HIV/AIDS prevention and control measures, the introduction and promotion of new measures for AIDS prevention and control and the experience and results obtained to the countries of the Belt and Road Initiative should be based on the characteristics of the HIV/AIDS epidemic in other countries. We should explore strategies and measures suitable for each country's national conditions and specific application environment, comprehensively study and analyze whether the prevention and control measures are suitable for the country's actual needs of HIV/AIDS prevention and control, and do a good job of policy advocacy to promote the adoption of such measures.

14.2 Risks of HIV/AIDS and Principles of Its Prevention and Control

14.2.1 Risk Assessment

Since 1981, HIV/AIDS has gradually spread globally, with significant changes in the geographical transmission routes of the epidemic and in the populations affected. In the early 1980s, that is, the early HIV/AIDS epidemic, AIDS cases were reported mainly from economically developed countries in North America and Europe. But in the middle and late 1980s, HIV began to spread in Africa and Asia. Over the past 40 years, the understanding of the risks of HIV epidemic has become increasingly comprehensive and clear, which is conducive to the development of effective and targeted measures for HIV prevention and control.

From the macro level, the HIV epidemic is actually a comprehensive reflection of social problems. Firstly, there is a change in epidemic risk areas, and the development of the HIV/AIDS epidemic in Asia is relatively late to the HIV/AIDS outbreak in Africa. In the 1980s, Thailand was the first country to receive attention. Because of its flourishing sex industry, a high HIV prevalence was found among sex workers in northern Thailand in 1989, followed by a peak in the epidemic among their male clients and housewives. During the same period, HIV/AIDS spread rapidly in large and medium-sized cities in some areas of Myanmar, Cambodia, and India, and then gradually to rural areas. Asia soon became the fastest-growing new epidemic center after Africa. The epidemic in China started in rural areas and spread to cities year by year. The second is the change in the routes of transmission. In the early HIV/AIDS epidemic, AIDS cases in developed countries in the United States and Europe were mainly caused by male–male sex, injecting drug users sharing syringes and hemophiliacs using HIV-contaminated anti-hemophilia globulin factors. With the concern for blood safety and the adoption of corresponding measures, the transmission of HIV through blood and blood products has been controlled, while drug injection and sexual transmission have become the main routes of transmission, and the proportion of heterosexual sexual transmission is gradually increasing. Heterosexual transmission has been the main route of HIV transmission in African countries. In Asia, there are mainly two epidemic patterns. One is heterosexual transmission, mainly in Thailand, India, and Cambodia. The other is mainly spread by injecting drug use, which gradually evolves into the coexistence of injecting drug use and heterosexual sexual transmission, mainly existing in Myanmar, Malaysia and some parts of China. In recent years, the increasing prevalence of HIV transmission through sex has been accompanied by the change of people's sexual concepts, mobility of people, social changes, especially the development of mobile information technology. The large population mobility and the wide application of new dating software provide more opportunities for sexual promiscuity. Out-of-wedlock, noncommercial and occasional sexual behaviors are another way of HIV transmission through sex. In today's society, with the development of new media, frequent information exchange and accelerated pace of life, this way, the main route of transmission of HIV epidemic is more secretive and difficult to control. The phenomenon of male–male sexual behavior has become more and more prominent, and has become one of the main driving forces of HIV transmission through sex in China's large and medium-sized cities and major countries in the Asia-Pacific region. The third is the change of high-risk populations. The number and proportion of HIV infections among sex workers and MSM are increasing. Effective prevention and treatment measures and strategies for these two high-risk populations are not yet ready, especially in the developing countries of the Belt and Road initiative, alternative, economical and effective measures and strategies are still very limited.

From the professional and technical point of view, AIDS is a serious infectious disease with its unique characteristics, the technical measures for its prevention and control are by far the most difficult for mankind. The asymptomatic incubation period of HIV infection is long, 8–10 years on average, which makes the diagnosis of HIV infection difficult. It is estimated that about 30% of HIV-infected people in China have not yet been diagnosed and continue to unknowingly transmit HIV. The dominant route of transmission in HIV/AIDS epidemic in China is sexual behavior, which is sensitive, complex, and difficult to control. In recent years, some new technologies for HIV prevention have emerged, and although they provides new options for controlling the sexual transmission of HIV, none of them can fundamentally solve the problem of sexual transmission of HIV. From the perspective of the basic principle of infectious disease control, no matter from the source of infection and transmission route, or from vulnerable population, an effective preventive technical measure must achieve adequate coverage at the social level so as to achieve the goal of controlling the epidemic.

In terms of molecular epidemiology, with the widespread use of highly active antiretroviral therapy (HAART) for HIV/AIDS all over the world, the occurrence of drug resistance and the prevalence of drug-resistant strains have followed. Due to the high variability of HIV virus and the high replication rate in human body, hundreds of millions of progeny viruses can be produced in infected individuals every day. Studies have shown that resistant strains can develop within weeks of treatment with a single drug or a combination of several drugs. Drug-resistant strains can even show up in cases that are not treated with such drugs, and replace the drug-sensitive strains as the dominant strains when treatment begins. Moreover, drug-resistant strains can further spread from person to person. Some studies have shown that subtype O of HIV-1 is naturally resistant to non-nucleotide reverse transcriptase inhibitors, subtype F is less sensitive to non-nucleotide reverse transcriptase inhibitors, subtype G is less sensitive to proteases than other subtypes, and mutations associated with antiprotease inhibitors tend to occur in those infected with non-B subtypes. Since most of the drugs currently used for HIV/AIDS treatment, such as nucleoside and non-nucleoside reverse transcriptase inhibitors and protease inhibitors, are designed and developed based on HIV-1 subtype B strains prevalent in Western countries, when these antiviral drugs are used against non-B subtypes prevalent worldwide, especially in developing countries, the actual therapeutic effect must be taken into account. The natural resistance of infected persons without antiviral treatment and the drug resistance that occurs after antiviral treatment are the current focus of attention.

14.2.2 Principles of Prevention and Control

Effective interventions to prevent HIV mainly target the three HIV transmission routes and reduce the incidence of new infections. The effectiveness of publicity and education on mastering relevant knowledge and raising awareness of prevention is obvious, but the effectiveness of publicity and education alone in reducing new HIV infections is limited. Publicity and education are mainly aimed at the vast majority of healthy people in society who have not had high-risk behaviors, and is effective in preventing high-risk behaviors, but for those who have high-risk behaviors, for example, injection drug users, MSM with unsafe sexual behavior, and sex workers, it has limited effectiveness, and must be combined with other more effective behavioral interventions.

For the prevention of sexual transmission of HIV, promoting and advocating safe sexual behavior is an important measure. Avoiding unsafe sex and always using a condom correctly for each sexual behavior is the most effective and economical way to prevent HIV infection through sexual transmission. In the 1990s, the HIV epidemic caused by prostitution and whoring was the main route of HIV transmission in Thailand and Cambodia. Their governments implemented a 100% condom policy in recreational places nationwide, which effectively controlled the HIV/AIDS epidemic. According to estimates by the Joint United Nations Programme on HIV/AIDS (UNAIDS) and the World Health Organization (WHO), Thailand's 100% condom using policy has prevented about two million HIV infections.

On the basis of summing up the experience of other countries and taking into account China's actual situation, China has adopted a comprehensive strategy of both drug control and HIV prevention. On the one hand, compulsory drug rehabilitation, community drug rehabilitation, and MMT are taken as win–win strategies and measures for drug control and HIV epidemic control so that these measures can complement each other. On the other hand, the implementation of MMT and clean needle program, with different emphasis in urban and rural areas, has produced better results. Despite the relatively late implementation of such measures in mainland China, progress has been rapid, and it has now become one of the countries with the largest number of MMT clinics and patients in the world, thereby effectively curbing the spread of drugs and the HIV epidemic caused by drug use.

In the 1990s, voluntary counseling and testing (VCT) was proposed as a strategy to find HIV infection and reduce its spread as a source of infection, with more emphasis on the voluntary testing right of infected people and respect for their voluntary choice. In 2006, on the basis of VCT, the CDC proposed a new strategy of provider-initiated HIV testing and counseling (PITC). Taking HIV test as a routine examination and playing down its particularity are conducive to finding more infected people and reducing social discrimination against HIV infection. It has played a great role in promoting HIV test and maximizing the detection of HIV infected people.

The primary strategy to prevent mother-to-child transmission of HIV is to prevent HIV infection in women of childbearing age, take HIV testing during pregnancy and parturition in women of childbearing age, apply antiviral drugs to pregnant and parturient women who have been infected with HIV, and provide comprehensive care and support for HIV-infected women and families, which greatly reduces mother-to-child transmission of HIV. With the price reduction and widespread use of antiviral drugs, a wide range of developing countries have implemented maternal and infant antiviral blocking work. In China, Southeast Asia (Thailand), and most countries in Africa, efforts to prevent mother-to-child transmission of HIV have been effective in reducing newborn HIV infections.

With the expansion of HIV treatment coverage, the mortality rate has significantly decreased and the number of new infections has remained stable, but it is still some way from the 2020 target proposed by UNAIDS (In 2016, the United Nations Political Declaration on Ending AIDS stated that Member States of the United Nations should commit themselves to reducing new HIV infections to fewer than 500,000 globally by 2020, reducing AIDS-related deaths to fewer than 500,000 globally by 2020, and ending the AIDS threat by 2030.). Combining behavioral and biomedical approaches and measures to control new HIV infections requires exploring the use of antiviral drugs for pre-exposure prophylaxis (PrEP) and post-exposure prophylaxis (PEP) based on the existing strategies including publicity and education, condom promotion, HIV testing and counseling, and antiviral treatment, so as to reduce the spread of HIV and control new HIV infections. PrEP is a preventative measure used to prevent HIV infection by taking antiviral drugs for those who are not yet infected with HIV but at risk of infection. PEP is a set of services that provide targeted prevention measures to individuals who are exposed and at risk of HIV infection in order to avoid HIV infection. At present, the strategy of PrEP and PEP has been developed in many countries, with guidelines issued by the United States, the European Union and the World Health Organization. However, in China, this strategy have not been widely recognized by the whole society, and the acceptance of the target population is still very limited. While there is sufficient evidence of the effectiveness and safety of PrEP and PEP and their significant effect on reducing new HIV infections, at the implementation level, the desired effect depends on the awareness of service providers and target populations about the strategy; the effective coordination of disease prevention and control institutions, medical institutions and community organizations to provide comprehensive, high-quality, and effective services; whether the patients have sufficient ability to pay, to maintain medication compliance, and to be regularly followed up and tested; whether progress can be made in the registration of drugs and whether the supply channels remain open, etc.

14.3 Cases of HIV/AIDS Prevention and Control

Experience and Effectiveness of MMT in Response to HIV Transmission by Injecting Drug Use in China

1. Overview

In 2006, most injecting drug users in China had high-risk behaviors of HIV infection such as sharing syringes and sexual promiscuity, resulting in a high rate of HIV infection ranging from 6.7% to 13.4% among them. The positive rate of HIV antibody once exceeded 20% in some regions with severe drug abuse in China, mainly distributed in Sichuan, Xinjiang, Guangxi, and Hunan, reaching as high as 69.7%, and the proportion of shared syringe was 46.8% on average. Therefore, in view of the situation of drug addiction in China (mainly heroin addiction), especially the situation of intravenous heroin addiction, drug treatment and behavioral intervention for heroin addicts are key tasks in the prevention and treatment of HIV infections and drug control.

According to the *China Drug Control Report 2011* released by the National Narcotics Control Commission, by the end of 2010, there were 15.445 million registered drug addicts nationwide, including 1.065 million heroin addicts, accounting for 69%, and 214,000 new heroin abusers were found in 2010. According to the *National Annual Report on Comprehensive HIV/AIDS Prevention and Control Data and Information* in 2011, the estimated monthly number of drug addicts was about 744,050, of which 361,973 were receiving HIV high-risk behavior intervention. The World Health Organization (WHO) pointed out that drug treatment should include drug therapy and psychosocial intervention. Methadone maintenance treatment (MMT) is one of the drug replacement therapies, which aims to help drug addicts to get rid of drug addiction, reduce diseases and deaths caused by drug abuse and high-risk behaviors related to drug abuse, improve their health status and quality of life, and provide them with relevant services so as to make them achieve physical and mental health as much as possible and obtain high level of social welfare and benefits [8]. MMT, as an effective means of treating opioid abuse, requires drug users to go to a designated place every day and take a certain dose of methadone orally under the supervision of a healthcare worker, thereby reducing the use of illegal drugs and related risk behaviors.

MMT was first used in New York in the 1960s for injecting drug users to control heroin addicts' cravings, and was aimed at social recovery rather than complete withdrawal. Since the 1980s, with the spread of the HIV/AIDS epidemic among drug users, MMT has been given new significance and content in "harm reduction" because it can reduce the risk behaviors associated with injecting drug use (sharing needles, cleaning needles together), and reduce unsafe sex, which in turn reduces reduce the chance of HIV infection [9]. In 2006, the Society for the Aid and Rehabilitation of Drug Abuser, Hong Kong launched the Sparks Action Program to provide services for HIV-infected patients to take methadone to reduce their chances of further transmission of HIV.

Based on the feasibility studies of MMT and international experience in MMT, in order to prevent the spread of HIV among injecting drug users and control drug abuse among heroin addicts, in February 2003, the Ministry of Health, the Ministry of Public Security and the State Food and Drug Administration jointly issued the *Notice on the Issuance of Interim Program of Pilot Work on Community Drug Maintenance Treatment for Heroin Addicts*. In March–June 2004, the first 8 MMT clinics were established in Yunnan, Guizhou, Sichuan, Guangxi, and Zhejiang [10].

2. Prevention and Control Strategies and Measures

China's Interim Program of Pilot Work on Community Drug Maintenance Treatment for Heroin Addicts stipulates that in general, there is only clinic that performs community MMT services in each county (city) administrative area, which is set up in the city or county disease prevention and control institution or medical institution. Conditions for drug users to be enrolled for methadone maintenance treatment: (1) heroin addicts who are still addicted to heroin after repeated drug treatment; (2) those who have undergone compulsory drug rehabilitation for twice or rehabilitation through labor for more than once; (3) over the age of 20; (4) local residents with a fixed residence; (5) with full capacity for civil conduct. Heroin addicts infected with HIV can be enrolled to receive MMT under conditions 4 and 5. According to the National Annual Report on Comprehensive HIV/AIDS Prevention and Control Data and Information in 2017, drug maintenance treatment has been extended to 762 clinics in 28 provinces (municipalities or autonomous regions), providing stable treatment to about 140,000 drug users. Community drug maintenance treatment has contributed to the control of drug abuse and HIV prevention and control in China, and has been recognized and supported by the society.

Because MMT can reduce drug use, drug-related social crimes and HIV epidemic caused by drug use, promote the recovery of individual and social functions of drug users, and contribute to the construction of a harmonious society, it has become the most important measure to control HIV epidemic among drug users in China. With the development of MMT in China, it has become one of the important strategies to prevent and control the spread of HIV through injection drug use. A large amount of evidence shows that the effectiveness of MMT is mainly reflected in the following aspects: **The first is to reduce drug use.** By taking methadone orally every day, drug users can reduce their cravings for heroin, suppress the euphoria that accompanies heroin use, suppress withdrawal symptoms, reduce heroin use, and thus reduce high-risk drug abuse behaviors such as needle sharing. **The second is to reduce high-risk sexual behavior.** Most injecting drug users have heterosexual sex, and in addition to sharing needles and other high-risk drug use behaviors, drug users can transmit HIV to their sexual partners through sexual intercourse. In addition to increasing condom use, MMT can reduce the number of high-risk sexual partners. **The third is to reduce the spread of HIV.** Drug users can infect or transmit HIV through sharing syringes or having sex with others, and preventing HIV transmission among drug users is an important purpose of drug treatment. The new HIV infection rate of MMT patients in China dropped from an average of 0.95% in 2006 to an average of 0.42% in 2010 [11]. **The fourth is to reduce heroin-related deaths.** It reduces deaths from heroin overdoses, infections with HIV and hepatitis C through syringe-sharing or high-risk sex. The fifth is to restore social and family functions. One of the basic purposes of MMT is to restore the social and family functions of patients, which include employment, residence, marriage, interpersonal relationship, and social support. The changes in social functions of drug users cannot be achieved in a short time because they need to change their social networks.

Since the initiation of community MMT and clean needle program in China in 2004, an average of about 200,000 drug users per year have participated in these two targeted control measures. After more than a decade of prevention and control practice, China has basically controlled the HIV epidemic among drug users. The incidence of new HIV infections among drug users with MMT dropped from 1% in 2006 to 0.07% in 2017, basically eliminating the occurrence of new HIV infections in these populations. The proportion of newly reported HIV infections through injecting drug use dropped from 44.2% in 2005 to less than 4% in 2017. The absolute number of newly diagnosed HIV-infected drug users per year dropped from a peak of about 16,000 in 2008 to about 4000 in 2017. Although injecting drug use is no longer the main route of HIV transmission in China, the two measures of MMT and clean needle program must be continued.

3. Summary of Experiences

After years of exploration and practice, the experiences in community MMT can be summarized as follows:

1. Proper positioning of MMT clinics. MMT has two main orientations: withdrawal of drug addiction and long-term maintenance. Patients in maintenance-targeted clinic treatment are 30% less likely to drop out of treatment within 1 year than those in clinic treatment targeted at withdrawal of drug addiction. When the orientation of clinic treatment shifted from "withdrawal" to "maintenance," patients' risk of dropping out of treatment after 3 years of treatment can be reduced by a third. Reasonable treatment orientation is essential for patients to stay in treatment.

2. Appropriate MMT costs. The costs borne by drug users have an important impact on participation in and adherence to MMT. The majority of drug users have a relatively poor financial situation and affordability due to long-term drug use, and low-cost or free MMT can make it easier for drug users to stay in treatment. Studies have shown [12] that providing free treatment to drug users can significantly prolong their stay in treatment, even if they have never received treatment before or are reluctant to receive treatment, and many enrolled patients continue to adhere to treatment after stopping free treatment. Qualitative studies conducted in Guangdong Province in China have found that reducing treatment costs in economically backward areas can improve clinic visits. Most MMT clinics in China charge fees appropriately, generally about 10 RMB, and adopt certain incentive methods. Compared with being completely free, it is more able to make patients attach importance to treatment and maintain their adherence to treatment.
3. Individualized MMT regimen and dose. The results of 21 MMT projects showed that the retention rates of short-term and long-term follow-up in the high-dose group (60–100 mg/day) were 1.36 and 1.62 times higher than those in the low-dose group (<60 mg/day), respectively. The key to maintaining the effectiveness of treatment is not the dose, but whether the dose is appropriate for each patient treated. China has proposed that the dosage of MMT should be individualized to ensure the treatment effect and reduce adverse reactions.
4. Proper allocation and quantity of MMT clinics. A study on influencing factors of MMT services for opioid addicts in Dehong Prefecture, Yunnan Province, found that long distance from the clinic, long travel time, and inconvenient transportation would limit the patients' use of MMT services. Therefore, in some provinces (autonomous regions) in China, such as Yunnan, Guangdong, Guangxi and Sichuan, a lot of MMT clinics are located in counties and rural areas. As drug users in rural areas are relatively dispersed, with vast geographical areas and inconvenient transportation, mobile MMT points and service points are promoted in rural areas to ensure the accessibility of MMT services.
5. Social support services provided at MMT clinics. Among the first eight MMT clinics in China, the maintenance treatment rate of the MMT clinic in Gejiu, Yunnan Province is the highest, with a maintenance rate of 84% and 65% at 6 months and 12 months, respectively, mainly due to the timely psychological counseling and intervention for drug users at the beginning of clinic treatment. MMT alone cannot solve all the problems of opioid addicts and additional psychosocial interventions are needed to improve treatment effect. Counseling and contingency management are the two most commonly used psychosocial interventions. Social support service activities are conducive to improving the relevant social behavioral charac-

teristics of drug users and making patients to stay in treatment. Drug addicts who have timely access to clinic care, family support, and assistance are able to stay in treatment for a longer period of time, and supportive services such as employment guidance, psychotherapy, and care are conducive to long-term maintenance of treatment.

Progress of Strategies and Measures for HIV Counseling and Testing in China

1. Summary

China's HIV counseling and testing strategies have undergone the stages of counseling, voluntary counseling and testing (VCT), provider-initiated HIV testing and counseling (PITC), and expanded testing [13]. Through the implementation of VCT, PITC, and expanded testing strategies, the number of HIV tests in 2018 reached 240 million, and 149,000 new infections were detected, an increase of 20.0% and 10.5% over 2017, respectively, and the reported detection rate reached 69.3%.

VCT can change unsafe sex, thereby reducing the risk of HIV transmission is an important measure to prevent HIV. Since 2003, China has initiated VCT work, and by the end of 2017, there were more than 10,000 consulting and testing sites nationwide. VCT has played an important role in the detection of HIV infection. In 2017, the number of HIV infections detected by VCT accounted for about 27% of the total number of newly reported HIV infections that year [14]. Moreover, the infected people detected by VCT are at an earlier stage of infection than those detected in medical institutions, which is more conducive to reducing the occurrence of new infections.

In order to strengthen the prevention and control of HIV infection, expand the coverage of HIV testing and counseling, so that more people can get tested for HIV and thus receive relevant treatment and prevention services, in response to the problem that HIV infection is difficult to find, in 2007, on the basis of voluntary counseling and testing (VCT), WHO proposed provider-initiated HIV testing and counseling (PITC), as a supplement to a variety of HIV detection strategies, and suggested that PITC should be carried out in all medical institutions in areas where the epidemic is widespread. Compared with VCT, in the PITC strategy, the word order of testing and counseling has been reversed to emphasize testing rather than counseling, reflecting the importance of testing to find HIV-infected persons. The publication of PITC guidelines and their adoption by countries further advanced the global HIV testing effort, helping to achieve the first 90% of UNAIDS' "three 90%" strategy, that is, 90% of those infected know their infection status. Beginning in 2011, in the 12th Five-Year Plan, China has taken maximizing the detection of HIV infections as one of its main prevention and treatment strategies.

The number of HIV tests conducted by medical institutions every year accounts for about 60% of the total number of people tested in China, and the number of HIV-infected people found accounts for more than 50% [15].

2. Prevention and Control Strategies and Measures

1. Counseling: In 1983–1995, the early years of the HIV epidemic, limited by the low level of localization of HIV diagnostic reagents and the high price of imported products, HIV testing in China was mainly carried out in epidemic prevention and quarantine institutions, mainly with suspected HIV patients found in medical institutions, drug abusers, sex workers and their clients, STD patients, MSM, and other related high-risk populations and entry–exit populations. It was extremely limited in number, scope, and object of testing. Some local governments were even concerned about the negative impact of the increase in the number of infections detected on local economic and social development. For those found to be infected with HIV, due to the lack of antiviral drugs, only a "symptomatic treatment" strategy focusing on controlling opportunistic infections can be adopted. Medical workers can only provide psychological comfort, family life guidance and medical follow-up observation to HIV-infected persons and their families based on their knowledge.
2. VCT: It is the process in which individuals can make their own choices about whether or not to be tested for HIV after counseling, and it stresses that the decision must be made by the individual and ensures that the testing process is secretive. The core of VCT is to provide patients with pretest counseling, post-test counseling and referral services (epidemiological investigation, behavioral intervention, antiviral therapy, comprehensive care and services) by professional counselors with strict confidentiality of patients' personal information. In 2003, after the Chinese government announced its "Four Frees and One Care" policy, providing free antiretroviral therapy to all people living with HIV (PLWH), free voluntary counseling and testing, free prevention of mother-to-child transmission services, free schooling for children orphaned or otherwise affected by HIV/AIDS, and economic assistance to households of PLWH, VCT as the main HIV detection strategy has been widely promoted. However, in the implementation process, due to too much emphasis on "willingness," the "labeling" of infected persons, the high demand for comprehensive quality of counselors, the lack of initiative of counselors in work, and the equating of "anonymity" with "confidentiality" in practice, it plays a very limited role in detecting infected people and in high-risk behavior interventions.
3. PITC strategy: It is initiated by medical workers in medical facilities to offer HIV testing and counseling to patients. The policy is based on the principle of "informed consent." Medical workers will do their routine work if the patient does not refuse, so they can make full use of existing

medical resources to expand the coverage of HIV testing and counseling. The main purpose of this approach is to allow medical workers to help patients make decisions or to provide information to medical services that need to know the HIV infection status of patients. Patients learn about their HIV infection status in a regular way of receiving medical services, which provides more opportunities for timely access to diagnosis, treatment, care, and prevention services. Compared with VCT, PITC has the advantages of better acceptability, higher HIV detection rate, better early detection of infected persons, and cost-effectiveness. Compared with VCT, PITC has higher requirements for counseling skills, with greater emphasis on promoting behavioral change, conducting risk assessment, and providing psychological support. PITC, on the other hand, has simplified and targeted counseling requirements, with a focus on testing and referrals, and an emphasis on informing results and providing follow-up support services such as treatment and care. Medical facilities have more opportunities to contact PLWH and are an important platform for detecting people living with HIV/AIDS. Carrying out PITC in medical facilities can expand the coverage of HIV testing and counseling, improve the detection rate of HIV infection, improve the intervention and assistance system, and enable patients to get effective treatment and intervention. The implementation of PITC strategy contributes to the detection of infected persons.

In recent years, with the change of HIV epidemic situation in China, more and more people living with HIV/AIDS are reported by medical institutions. PITC reduces the informing and counseling before and after testing, leaving the patients free to choose. However, infected patients detected in medical facilities are often incurably ill patients, who are difficult to treat and have high mortality, thus limiting the role of PITC in controlling new infections and viral transmission.

4. Expanded testing strategy: The main goal is to expand the coverage of testing, maximize the detection of infected people, focus on the detection of key populations, and expand to other populations. Clinical treatment and mathematical model studies suggest that, although it is difficult to reduce HIV infection rate due to behavioral patterns, for people living with HIV, timely diagnosis, high-quality medical care, coupled with adherence to effective antiviral treatment, can reduce the chance of secondary transmission, reduce the infectivity of each high-risk behavior, prolong life expectancy, reduce the impact on personal life, and reduce the risk of AIDS-related diseases and death. If this strategy reaches a certain level of coverage among HIV-infected populations, the incidence of HIV will decline and, and if it can last for decades, it is expected to curb the HIV epidemic. From the perspective of health economics, it has good cost-effectiveness in high or low HIV prevalence areas, among different high-risk populations and in prevention of mother-to-child transmission. "HIV testing and Treatment as

Prevention" has become an epochal milestone in global health policies on HIV/AIDS. In the United States, only one in every six adults was tested for HIV in the late 1980s. Through publicity and multiple ways to expand testing, the number of people tested has been increasing year by year, reaching 88% in 2012 and more than 90% in 2016. China has accumulated a lot of practical experience in promoting full HIV screening in hospitals, blood stations, and among pregnant and lying-in women. The launch of National HIV Counseling and Testing Month in 2018 further promotes the strategy of expanded HIV testing. The strategy of expanded HIV testing focuses on the establishment of rapid testing sites in towns, townships, communities, and social organizations. From the pilot experience of testing sites, it is increasingly effective in timely detection of HIV infection in rural areas and among MSM.

3. Summary of Experiences

HIV testing, the only means to detect PLWH, should be further strengthened. Especially in the current stage of expanding and improving the accessibility of antiviral treatment, it is necessary to carry out expanded testing according to law and in a scientific way, to adopt a comprehensive testing strategy, and to provide universally accessible, acceptable, and efficient testing services. Besides, it is urgent to strengthen social security and create a nondiscriminatory social environment.

1. Expand the coverage of publicity and education of HIV/AIDS prevention and control, and improve the public's awareness of self-health and responsibility.

   HIV/AIDS prevention and treatment also follow the principles and methods of "early intervention, early detection and early treatment." At present, "a large number of HIV-infected people having not been detected" remains a key constraint on the reduction of new infections and antiviral treatment and other prevention and treatment services. In China's 13th Five-Year Action Plan for Containment and Control of HIV/AIDS, "improving access to testing and counseling" is an important prevention and control measure. Providers of testing services (institutions and healthcare workers) should be fully aware of the importance of expanded testing for HIV prevention and control and for the promotion of population health.
2. Increase willingness to test for HIV and promote the utilization of testing services.

   The low willingness of the target population to HIV testing services is an important factor hindering detection of HIV infection at present.

Effective ways to address this problem include increased publicity, especially about HIV epidemic and testing content and institutions, so that more people can understand the importance of testing services, and reduce discrimination and increase social inclusion; accelerate the construction of inspection points and personnel capacity to provide fast, convenient, and accessible services to those in need; strengthen the cooperation between CDCs and social organizations, support qualified and capable community-based organizations to provide testing and proactive surveillance for the timely detection of new HIV infections; and inform spouses (sexual partners) of HIV-infected persons newly detected as early as possible, and encourage them to undergo HIV testing while taking personal protection.

3. Enrich HIV testing methods to improve the accessibility of testing services.

   On the basis of proper planning and construction of the network of HIV testing laboratories, take further targeted measures to strengthen combined testing strategies such as VCT, PITC, and testing with the participation of social organizations, strengthen pilot studies according to relevant policies, promote self-testing and community-testing methods, enrich testing service means, provide people with more service options, and increase the accessibility and acceptability of testing services through combinatorial and structured strategies and methods.

4. Advocate the "benefit principle" and promote the "one-stop" service of testing, detection, and timely treatment.

   Taking focusing on people's needs and benefiting service recipients as the main principle to mobilize people to participate in HIV testing, providing timely treatment and other healthcare services for the infected persons and patients found in the testing can help increase the effectiveness of testing mobilization, improve the willingness to HIV testing services, and meet the needs of the service recipients in an all-round way. China's "one-stop" service is one of the strategies for HIV prevention and control, and the "one-stop" services for TB and HIV control in some Southeast Asian and African countries are also recommended by UNAIDS.

5. Constantly innovate strategies and methods to cultivate the concept of "health first" among target populations.

   Advocate the ideas of "health conscious" and "the first wealth is health", and advocate the strategy of awareness of HIV testing results before sex and testing by peers among MSM and other target populations.

References

1. Health Topic: HIV/AIDS. http://www.chinacdc.cn/jkzt/crb/zl/azb/. Accessed 1 Oct 2020.
2. Subtypes of HIV. http://www.aids.org.cn/article-detail?id=3930. Accessed 25 Sep 2020.
3. Wang L. HIV/AIDS Prevention and Treatment. [M]. Beijing: Beijing Press, Beijing Publishing Group; 2009.
4. National Health Commission, PRC. Diagnosis of AIDS and HIV infection. http://www.nhc.gov.cn/wjw/s9491/201905/6430aa653728439c901a7340796e4723.shtml. Accessed 25 Sep 2020.
5. Pengqian F, Jiahui Z, Juan X. Definition and category of HIV/AIDS high-risk populations in China [J]. Chin J AIDS STD. 2006;5:470–1.
6. Zunyou W. Advances in HIV/AIDS prevention technology and control strategies [J]. Chin J Prevent Med. 2018;052(012):1204–9.
7. Zhenquan J. China's HIV/AIDS control strategy and analysis. Hangzhou: The Sixth International Conference on HIV/AIDS; 2019.
8. WHO, UNAIDS, UNODC. Evidence for action on HIV/AIDS and injecting drug use. Policy brief: reduction of HIV transmission through drug-dependence treatment. https://www.who.int/hiv/pub/advocacy/en/throughoutreachen.pdf. Accessed 25 Sep 2020.
9. Hall W, Mattick RP. Role of maintenance treatment in opioid dependence [J]. Lancet. 1999;353(9148):221–2.
10. Ministry of Health, Ministry of Public Security, State Food and Drug Administration. Circular on the Publication of Interim Program of Pilot Work on Community Drug Maintenance Treatment for Heroin Addicts. CDC [2006] No 37 Beijing, 2003.
11. Zunyou W. New realities and challenges facing China's HIV/AIDS prevention and treatment. Chin J Public Health. 2011;27(12):1505–7.
12. Kwiatkowski CF, Booth RE, Lloyd LV. The effects of offering free treatment to street-recruited opioid injectors [J]. Addiction. 2000;95(5):697–704.
13. Xi C. Strategies for expanding testing in the context of HIV antiviral treatment [J]. Chin J Prevent Med. 2018;52(12):1210–4.
14. National Center for AIDS/STD Control and Prevention/National Center for STD Control, China CDC. Annual Report on Comprehensive Prevention and Treatment of HIV/AIDS, STD and Hepatitis C in China (2017) [M]. Beijing: National Center for AIDS/STD Control and Prevention/National Center for STD Control, China CDC; 2018.
15. Zunyou W. China's achievements and challenges in fight against HIV/AIDS 1985–2015 [J]. Chin J Epidemiol. 2015;

Correction to: Prevention and Control of Infectious Diseases in BRI Countries

Weizhong Yang

Correction to: Prevention and Control of Infectious Diseases in BRI Countries https://doi.org/10.1007/978-981-33-6958-0

The original version of this book was unfortunately published with errors in the affiliation of book editor which has now been corrected in the copyright page, contributors list, chapters 1 and 14 to Chinese Academy of Medical Sciences & Peking Union Medical College, Chinese Preventive Medicine Association, The UN Consultative Committee on Life Science and Human Health (CCLH) of China Association of Science and Technology (CAST).

Chapter 6: Caption of figure 6.1, the first paragraph under section 6.1.1 Seasonal Influenza, reference 1. This has now been corrected and an erratum to this book has been published. The corrections can be found at https://doi.org/10.1007/978-981-33-6958-0_15.

The updated online version of the chapters can be found at
https://doi.org/10.1007/978-981-33-6958-0
https://doi.org/10.1007/978-981-33-6958-0_1
https://doi.org/10.1007/978-981-33-6958-0_6
https://doi.org/10.1007/978-981-33-6958-0_14

W. Yang (ed.), *Prevention and Control of Infectious Diseases in BRI Countries*,
https://doi.org/10.1007/978-981-33-6958-0_15

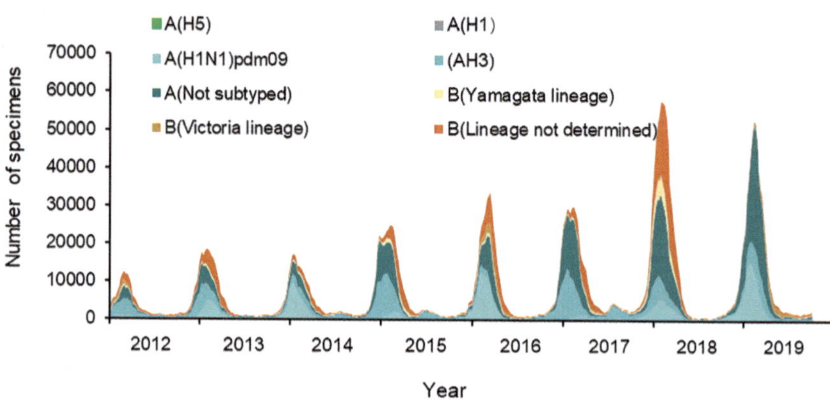

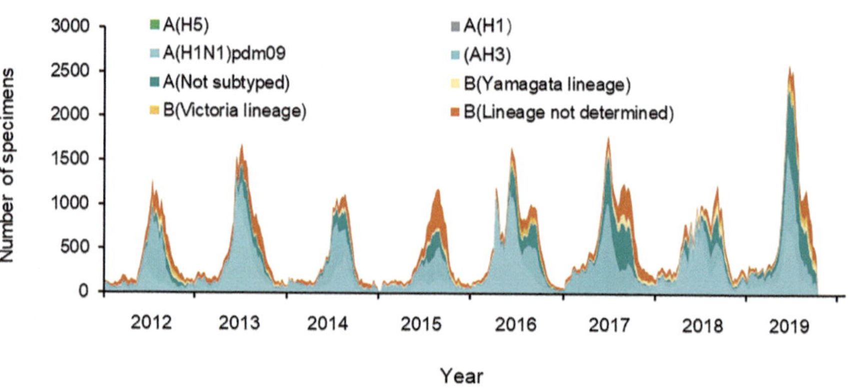

Fig. 6.1 Number of specimens positive for influenza by subtype in the Northern and Southern hemisphere from the 1st week of 2012 to the 40th week of 2019

GPSR Compliance

The European Union's (EU) General Product Safety Regulation (GPSR) is a set of rules that requires consumer products to be safe and our obligations to ensure this.

If you have any concerns about our products, you can contact us on ProductSafety@springernature.com

In case Publisher is established outside the EU, the EU authorized representative is:

Springer Nature Customer Service Center GmbH
Europaplatz 3
69115 Heidelberg, Germany

Batch number: 10370712

Printed by Printforce, the Netherlands